DERMATOLOGY

SERVET
CLINICAL GUIDE

ALLERGIES

Gustavo Machicote Goth

Plaza Antonio Beltrán Martínez n° 1, planta 8 - letra I
(Centro empresarial El Trovador)
50002 Zaragoza - Spain

First printing: May 2018

This book has been published originally in Spanish under the title:
Guía Servet de manejo clínico: Dermatología. Alergias
© 2018 Grupo Asís Biomedia, S.L.
ISBN Spanish edition: 978-84-17225-07-0

Translation:
Jason Willis-Lee
Review:
Lori Newman

ISBN: 978-84-17225-63-6
D.L.: Z 612-2018

Design, layout and printing:
Servet editorial - Grupo Asís Biomedia, S.L.
www.grupoasis.com
info@grupoasis.com

Servet is the publishing house of Grupo Asís

Warning:

Veterinary science is constantly evolving, as are pharmacology and the other sciences. Inevitably, it is therefore the responsibility of the veterinary surgeon to determine and verify the dosage, the method of administration, the duration of treatment and any possible contraindications to the treatments given to each individual patient, based on his or her professional experience. Neither the publisher nor the author can be held liable for any damage or harm caused to people, animals or properties resulting from the correct or incorrect application of the information contained in this book.

ACKNOWLEDGEMENTS

I would like to thank the AVEPA Group of Specialists in Dermatology (GEDA) for allowing me to work alongside so many friends within the field of dermatology. I also thank AVEPA for safeguarding the specialty and helping us to improve on a daily basis.

Thanks to Servet Publishing and the entire team for being such good collaborators.

Thanks to the owners of allergic pets, who are so patient with us.

And finally, thanks to my family, who endures my lengthy absences to study, communicate, and write.

DEDICATION

This book is dedicated to all those owners/friends of our patients who often befriend us as well; to so many of my colleagues who diligently strive to help our pets; and finally, to those dear cats and dogs that endure so much and ask only to be loved in return.

FOREWORD

It is my great pleasure to introduce this work by my colleague Gustavo Machicote, who has also been a close friend for over 15 years.

The book is aimed at veterinary clinicians and students, and its main purpose is to provide a useful and current tool to further and consolidate their knowledge in one of the most exciting and complex fields within veterinary dermatology: allergic diseases of pets.

The book is split into several chapters that tackle different facets of managing hypersensitive patients, ranging from diagnostic protocols to the most current treatments. It includes a magnificent collection of photographs that help to understand and follow the text; the result is an enjoyable and educational read each step of the way.

The reader gets an impression of authenticity and truth based on diligent clinical practice, together with marked scientific rigour that arises from tireless study.

Today, in the so-called "information era" where we are bombarded daily with enormous amounts of information, we should recognise works that probe beyond superficial description, in which the author tackles real-life

FOREWORD

clinical cases that are often absent from traditional texts or addressed only superficially. Against this backdrop, I believe it especially useful to provide a chapter on the veterinary surgeon's communication with owners of allergic patients. This is a persistent issue that all clinicians should improve upon, not only in the field of dermatology but in every veterinary discipline. In management of dermatological diseases, and more particularly in chronic cases such as those due to hypersensitivity, communication with the owner is the critical determinant of treatment success. Along these lines, the capacity for empathy and the effort dedicated to opening lines of communication with owners are vitally important.

To conclude, I would like to highlight the role of "paper" books and guides such as this one. Although veterinary training has been enormously diversified and enriched with information technology, and we are increasingly utilising online or virtual sources to supplement our training, it is a real pleasure for me to open a new dermatology book, dive into its pages, and inhale that "new book smell".

César L. Yotti
Skinpet Veterinary Dermatology Centre

PREFACE

When I received Grupo Asís' kind invitation to write this guide, I felt proud and enthusiastic about the proposal and the opportunity to write about a current hot topic in the field of small animal veterinary medicine, namely allergies.

At that time, I brainstormed and asked myself whether I was more interested in creating an academic reference work on the dermatology of skin allergies or a daily reference tool for my many colleagues who wrestle with diverse cases every day without the luxury to specialise in one particular topic.

This work includes knowledge I have acquired from evidence-based medicine, as well as the experience of my daily practice and that of my many fellow veterinary dermatologists.

A major revolution in the field of veterinary dermatology has occurred in the last few years, with the arrival of new drugs on the market and an increase in training opportunities offered by pharmaceutical companies and associations. We are in the midst of this revolution, which continues today. Thus, I feel that authoring a book today is more or less like purchasing technology. We know that new advances will occur soon, and we will have to stay up-to-date.

PREFACE

All medical specialities involve the treatment of diseases that may be more or less significant in the patient's life; while allergies are not immediately life-threatening, they do alter the pet–owner lifestyle and may transform the joy of owning a pet into the torment of very unpleasant, uncomfortable situations for both the animal and its owner. I have always believed that every small animal veterinary surgeon should experience having an allergic pet at home to be able to empathise with the client/owners whom we "educate" on therapy, which is not always easy to institute.

Allergic diseases in general must be managed therapeutically, meaning we seek to control rather than cure them. This means that the owner of an allergic pet is a very regular client who has to coexist with not only their pet but also their veterinary surgeon, who might also become a confidant about the disease. Our aim as therapists is always to try and manage the disease by minimising acute episodes and ensuring as few visits to the clinic as possible. This kind of disease requires greater empathy and stronger veterinary clinician–owner relationships than other more temporary diseases.

I hope that this management and diagnostic guide for the dermatology of allergies serves its purpose, which is simply to assist veterinary surgeons in treating these conditions on a daily basis.

Gustavo Machicote Goth
Dermapet. Veterinary Dermatology Service

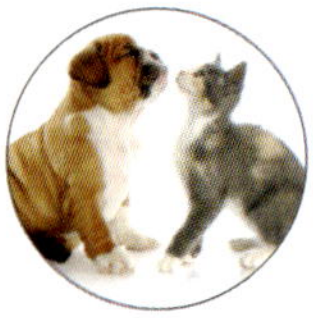

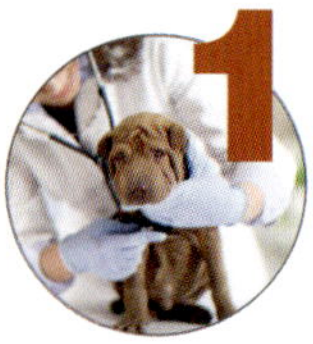

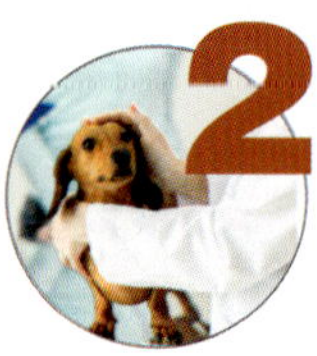

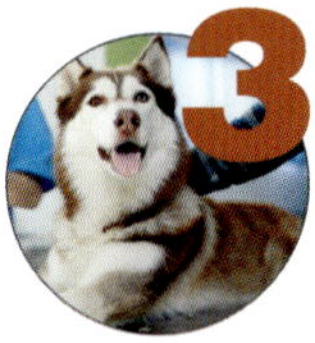

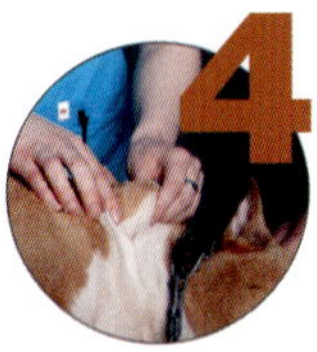

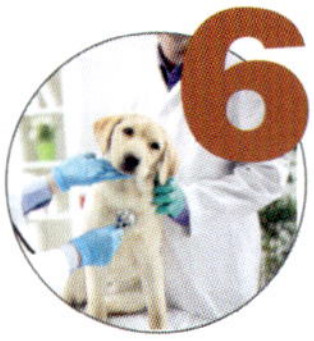

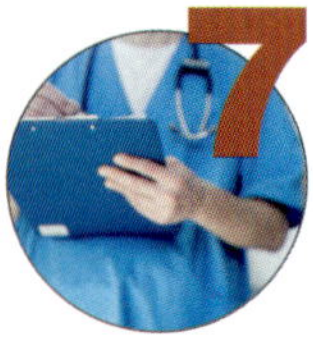

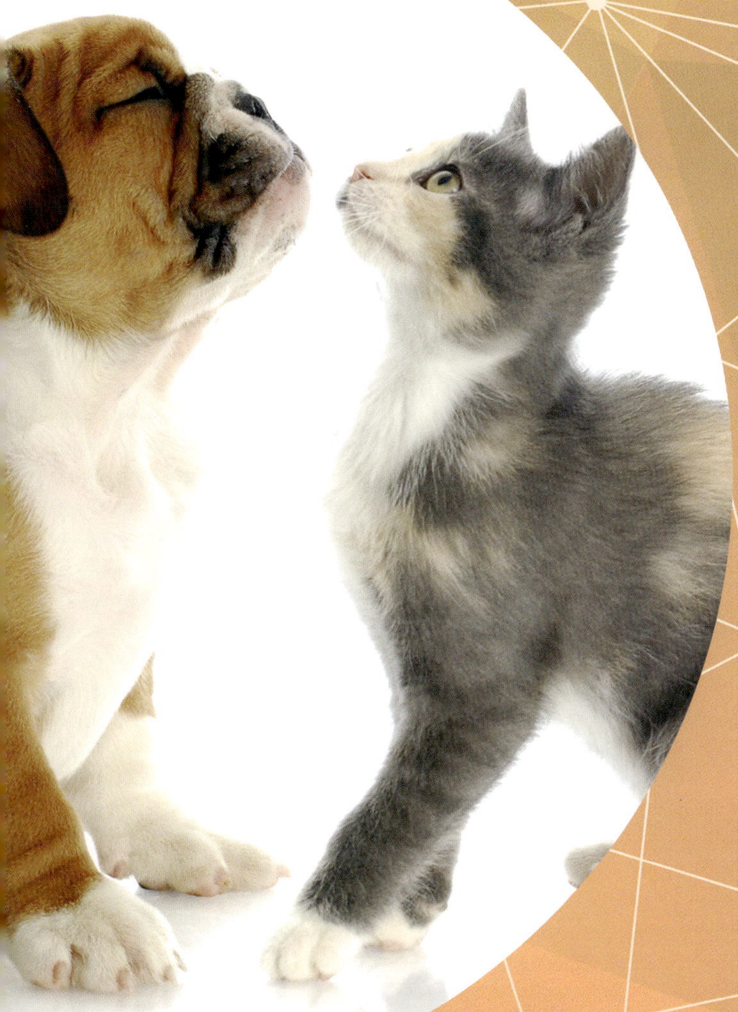

READ ME FIRST

READ ME FIRST

Dermatological conditions are among the most commonly seen in routine small animal practice. Pruritus is nearly always the most significant presenting complaint of the owner. It can vary in intensity depending on disease severity. This information is summarised in the table below (Fig. 1).

DEGREE OF PRURITUS	1–2	3–4	5–6	7–8	9–10
Clinical signs	Occasional scratching	Frequent scratching	Scratches most of the day but stops when distracted.	Stops eating or playing to scratch. Difficult to distract the animal.	Compulsive scratching all the time. Requires an Elizabethan collar.
Sequelae	No lesions observed	Mild excoriations	Excoriations, moist areas with intertrigo (from licking)	Excoriations, pyotraumatic dermatitis, intertrigo	Self-mutilation that leads to bleeding.
Owner	Almost imperceptible	Worse indoors than outdoors. Treatment as required.	Difficult to live with the animal. Requires treatment, sometimes topical.	Effective and systemic treatment. Owner is concerned.	Emergency treatment. Combination therapies. Desperate owners.

Figure 1. Degrees of pruritus.

This neuro-dermatological sensation, which can manifest in many ways, such as licking, scratching, chewing, shaking, and behavioural changes, is quite uncomfortable for both the patient and the owner.

> The principal sign of allergies is generally pruritus, and allergies are the most common primary complaint in specialty practice.

READ ME FIRST

The three most significant types of allergies by far are environmental, to food and to flea bites; together, these account for most of the cases of pruritus seen today.

Such diseases have long posed significant challenges, and they remain the obvious research target for many investigators and pharmaceutical companies because these problems threaten the coexistence of pets with their owners. In the last few years, a revolution has started in allergy diagnosis and therapy, and it is certain to continue.

In a short time, we have moved from a limited range of drug options, possibly due to poor knowledge of the aetiopathogenesis of the disease, to a much wider array of both diagnostic and treatment options. This is enabling resolution of clinical cases that until a short time ago could not be controlled or could be controlled only in ways that endangered the patient's health.

The veterinary profession has evolved significantly in the last few years and will continue to do so exponentially as clinicians become more specialised and owners become more aware of the diagnostic and therapeutic possibilities. Moreover, veterinary surgeons are increasingly cognisant of the complexity of this multifactorial disease and its genetic predispositions.

> Each individual suffers completely distinct signs and complications, despite having the same "disease".

In addition to the cat and dog having completely distinct hypersensitivities, the varied genetic profiles within the same species produce a huge variety of allergic signs. Genetic differences also alter drug responses, meaning that treatments must be tailored to each individual. The evolving discipline of pharmacogenetics addresses this issue.

Recently, the incidence of allergic diseases has increased significantly in both human and veterinary medicine. There are various theories that account for this increase, and research mainly from human medicine but with reference to veterinary medicine summarises these as follows:

1. **Environmental pollution hypothesis**
   Climate change and pollution of habitats and the environment affect both humans and animals. The increase in pets living indoors may have increased their exposure to certain allergens. This criterion is often considered for the diagnosis of allergies, mainly in dogs.

2. **Dietary alterations**
   The use of more additives and preservatives and, in some cases, incorrectly formulated diets may be related to the aetiopathogenesis of adverse food reactions (AFR). Intestinal inflammation in puppies caused by poor diet, parasites or viruses may induce intestinal permeability that exposes them to larger polypeptide chains that can induce future AFRs.

3. **Hygiene hypothesis**
   Excessive cleaning and avoidance of natural interaction with the environmental. This theory is quite well-documented in human medicine. However, veterinary medicine lacks scientific evidence to back this. It would be interesting to research the relationship between the very common parasite prevention and vaccination regimens for puppies and the increased incidence of allergy.

4. **Genetic factors**
   Allergic individuals continuing to breed can pose a problem. This is well-documented in veterinary medicine, where certain breeds have a much higher prevalence of allergic disease.

5. **Increased stress and smoking**
   Smoking might play a role for pets that live with smokers. Regarding stress, certain behavioural disorders may be expressed as anxiety and may exacerbate allergic signs. Sometimes there is a fine line between compulsive scratching because of allergies and stereotypy.

6. **Improved diagnosis**
Veterinary medicine has developed much better diagnosis of this group of diseases. However, genetic selection, often dependent on breeders, remains an outstanding issue. The selection of allergy-free breeding animals is extremely important and owners/breeders should assume this responsibility.

This section will conclude with a special section dedicated to cats.

Cats are increasingly popular pets, so veterinary clinicians are increasingly focused on feline medicine and catering to feline behaviour.

> Within both dermatology and allergy, the cat is quite distinct from the dog.

Cats are much more reserved in behaviour and much less "transparent" about allergy-induced skin discomfort. Pruritus often manifests in another way in cats; these may lick surreptitiously or while hiding. Lesions are also completely different from those in dogs. Feline treatments also vary, and veterinary surgeons will see new therapeutic options resources for this species in the near future.

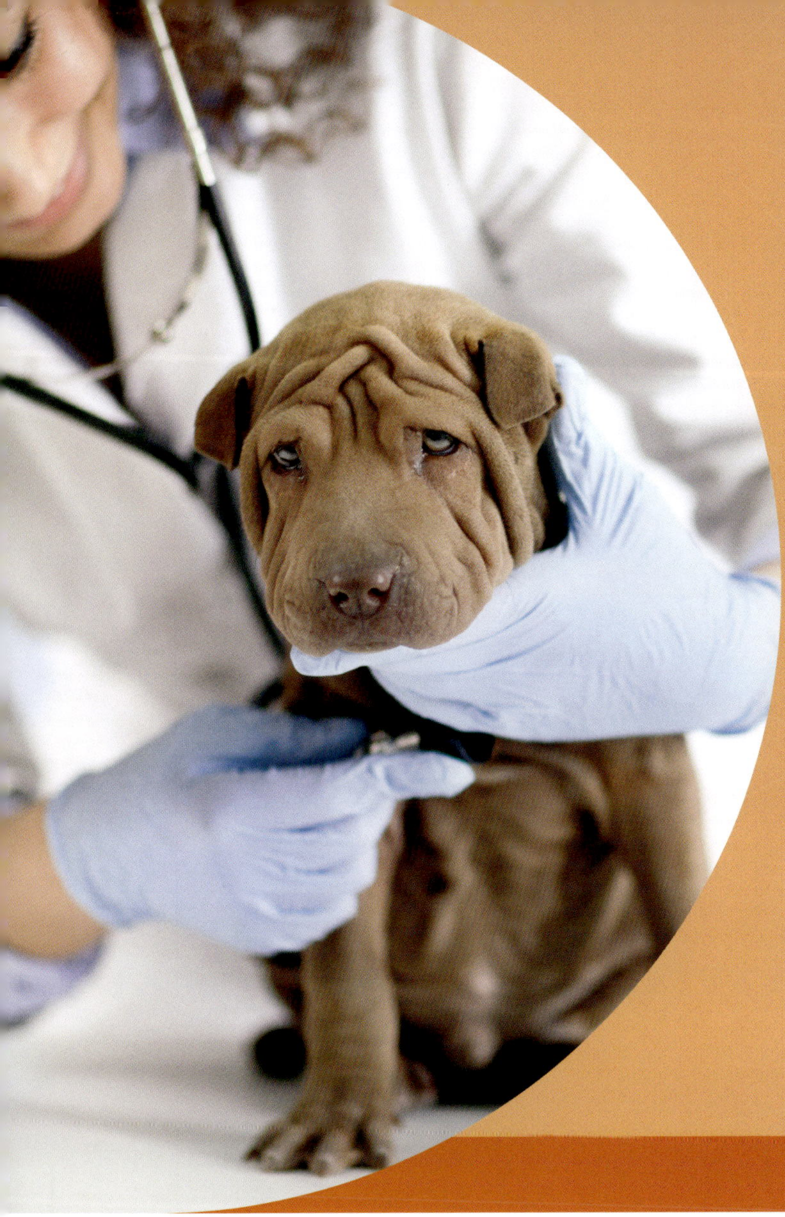

1

CLINIC CONSULTATION

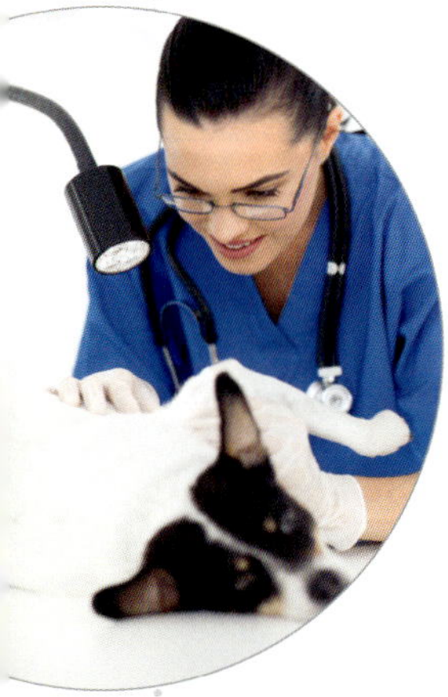

WHAT DOES THE OWNER
NOTICE FIRST?

When dealing with owners of allergic pets, the first aspect to consider is the type of pet–owner bond.
Owners that live in close confinement with their pets, for example, in a shared flat, are often very concerned as they also "suffer" their animal's illness. Owners with a less tight space (e.g. a home with a garden or a farm) or of completely outdoor animals may "witness" the clinical signs, but the impact of the condition on the coexistence with their pets will be minor.

Do not overlook prior experience that owners may have had when they notice the initial signs, whether from having had other affected animals or even a relative with the same disease.

The veterinary surgeon's professional approach must not be affected by the kind of owner, but our work is more effective if we adapt to their individual characteristics.

The aim is to resolve the patient's presenting complaint.

To achieve this, we must first earn their trust in order to maximise our therapeutic efficacy.

In the case of dogs, the first thing the owner observes is that their animal's normal activity is altered or interrupted by bouts of itching or licking. This is often accompanied by visible abnormalities on the skin such as erythema or alopecia (Fig. 1).

In cats, the problem differs slightly due to their much more reserved behaviour and their varied cutaneous reaction patterns. A cat owner may initially notice signs of miliary dermatitis or localised self-induced alopecia (Fig. 2). Facial lesions and eosinophilic reactions are generally less common, but in some cases much more notable, signs.

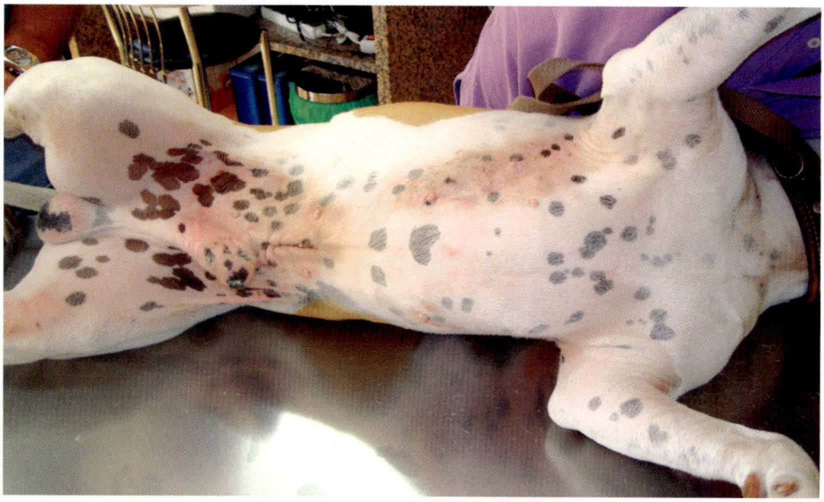

Figure 1. Initial signs of erythema in the ventral axillary and inguinal areas.

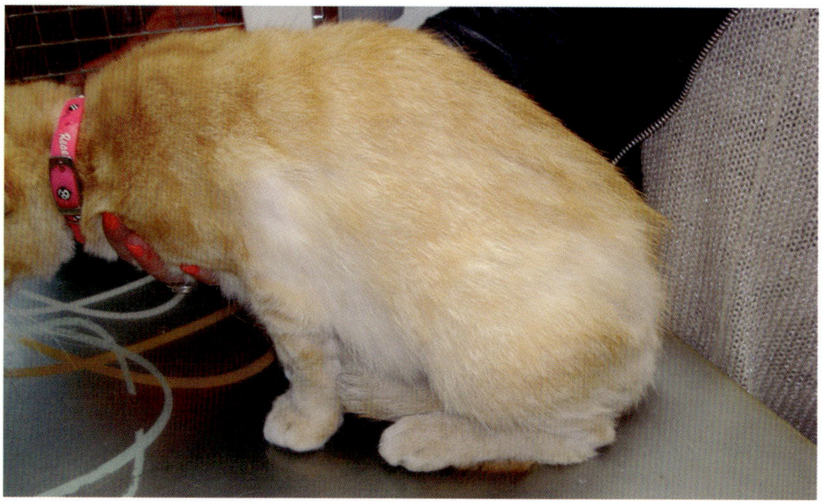

Figure 2. Focal self-induced alopecia in a cat. Note the areas of hypotrichosis.

<table>
<tr><th colspan="2">THE OWNER'S PERSPECTIVE</th></tr>
<tr><td>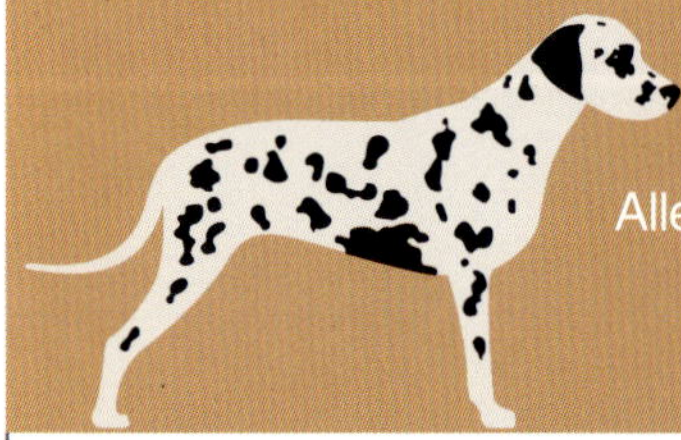 Allergic dog</td><td>Allergic cat 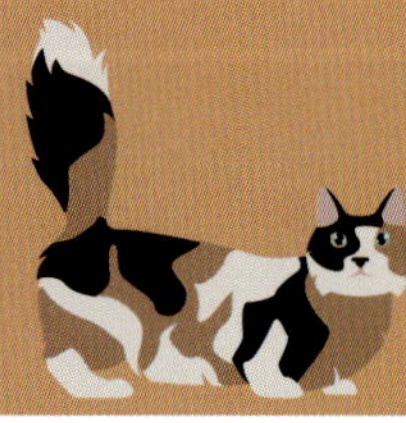</td></tr>
<tr><td colspan="2">It may be difficult to understand that allergy is a chronic disease requiring lifelong therapy.</td></tr>
<tr><td>They may seek second opinions in search of a definitive "cure".</td><td>They may neglect the importance of behavioural health in cats with allergy.</td></tr>
<tr><td>Pruritus appears uncomfortable for both the dog and family.</td><td>The aggressive reaction pattern of head and neck dermatitis can lead owners to despair.</td></tr>
<tr><td>They might not realise signs such as licking, chewing, shaking and rubbing are manifestations of pruritus.</td><td>They may think scratching does not occur because they do not see it (cats often scratch in hiding).</td></tr>
<tr><td>They may have difficulty understanding that pruritus is the sum of several causes exceeding a threshold.</td><td>They may believe that scratching is a normal part of grooming.</td></tr>
<tr><td>They may aspire to a pruritus score of 0 (on a scale from 0 to 10).</td><td>They may overlook the importance of environmental enrichment and the use of pheromones to reduce pruritus.</td></tr>
<tr><td>Alopecia may appear socially and aesthetically uncomfortable.</td><td>They may believe that self-induced alopecia is actually spontaneous hair loss (if they do not see the cat licking itself).</td></tr>
<tr><td colspan="2">If the animal is a long-haired breed, they may resist cutting the hair to optimise treatment.</td></tr>
<tr><td>It may be difficult for them to follow a hypoallergenic diet.</td><td>It may be difficult for them to commence a specific diet.</td></tr>
<tr><td>Bathing 2–3 times per week and offering a strict diet may appear labour-intensive and expensive.</td><td>It may be difficult for them to bathe and administer oral medicines to their cat.</td></tr>
<tr><td>They may not believe the animal has fleas because they do not see any.</td><td>They may not believe the animal could have fleas because the cat never leaves the house.</td></tr>
<tr><td colspan="2">They may not consider the role of the environment in treatment. It is important to avoid exposure to allergens and eliminate juvenile fleas.</td></tr>
</table>

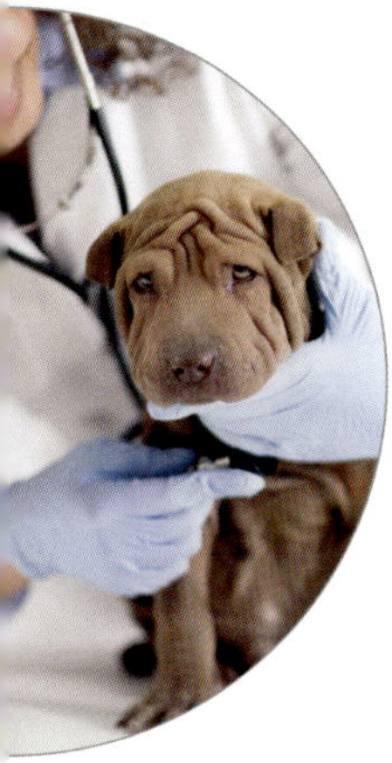

HISTORY
TO GUIDE DIAGNOSIS

Veterinary clinicians, including dermatologists, recognise that pruritus is undoubtedly the clinical sign that requires most attention within the field of dermatology. Given that allergies are the most common cause of pruritus, it is difficult to remain impartial during diagnosis.

To avoid mistakes, it is critical to follow a diagnostic algorithm that rules out all the differential diagnoses until only the possible allergy remains.

The most common allergic skin disease is atopic dermatitis (AD)/adverse food reaction (AFR) complex.

Diagnosis is generally based on the clinical signs and established criteria that confirm the disease with high specificity and sensitivity.

These criteria were established many years ago to critically evaluate clinical suspicions and were ultimately adapted by Favrot et al. They will be discussed in detail in the next chapter.

Certain owner comments in the history may jump out to suggest a possible allergy.

WHAT LEADS
TO CLINICAL SUSPICION OF ALLERGY?

OWNER COMMENTS THAT SUGGEST AN ALLERGY	
DOGS	CATS
Increased shaking of the head (ear pruritus).	*Vomits hairballs frequently.*
Licks and chews its paws a lot, mainly the front ones.	*There are bald spots but I do not see hair loss.*
Drags its bottom across the floor (anal pruritus).	*Grooms a lot, obviously very clean.*
Rubs its face against anything it can.	*The only thing that helps is that injection given occasionally.*
Its ears turn red after a walk.	*It is incredible how thoroughly my pet grooms.*
In addition to scratching, it also rolls a lot.	
Its bowel sounds are loud.	
Every time the pills are stopped, it starts scratching again.	

PREDISPOSING FACTORS

In dogs, research, diagnostic criteria, and clinical evidence and experience suggest these predisposing factors*:

- Living indoors.
- Genetic predisposition. Certain breeds have greater prevalence.
- Suffering from gastrointestinal disorders as a puppy (exposure to allergens due to permeable intestinal mucosa).
- Frequent exposure to mites and other allergens from a young age.

In cats, predisposing factors are:

- Hereditary predisposition. Certain breeds are more predisposed to eosinophilic granuloma complex (e.g. Norwegian Forest cat and some white-coated breeds).

* There is no strong scientific basis for these factors except the first one.

COMMON AND RARE CLINICAL SIGNS IN CATS AND DOGS

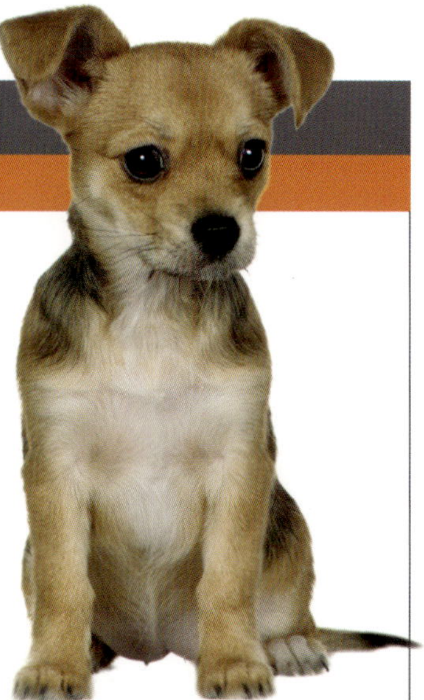

DOGS

COMMON CLINICAL SIGNS

- Pruritus with or without secondary lesions.
- Surface bacterial overgrowth (Fig. 3).
- *Malassezia* overgrowth.
- Recurrent pyoderma, a little deeper than the overgrowths.
- Occasional or recurrent otitis.
- Foot licking (Fig. 4).
- Anal pruritus.
- Erythema, mainly in the ears and axillary, and inguinal areas.
- Facial lesions, mainly around the eyes and lips.
- Alopecia, generally in a moth-eaten pattern.
- Gastrointestinal abnormalities, mainly bowel sounds and changes in the consistency of faeces.

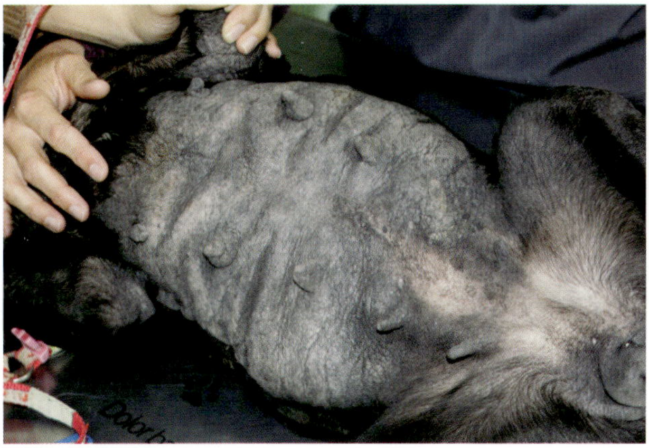

Figure 3. Chronic microbial overgrowth.

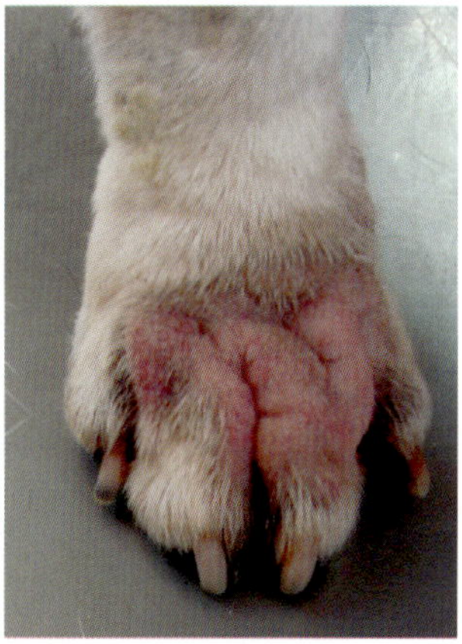

Figure 4. Dorsal foot affected by persistent licking.

RARE CLINICAL SIGNS

- Conjunctivitis.
- Rhinitis.
- Tracheobronchitis.
- Recurrent deep pyoderma (Fig. 5).
- Acral lick dermatitis.
- Severe gastrointestinal abnormalities.
- Recurrent angioedema and urticaria.
- Anal gland impaction.
  This may be common in some breeds.
- Onychomadesis.
- Perianal fistulae.

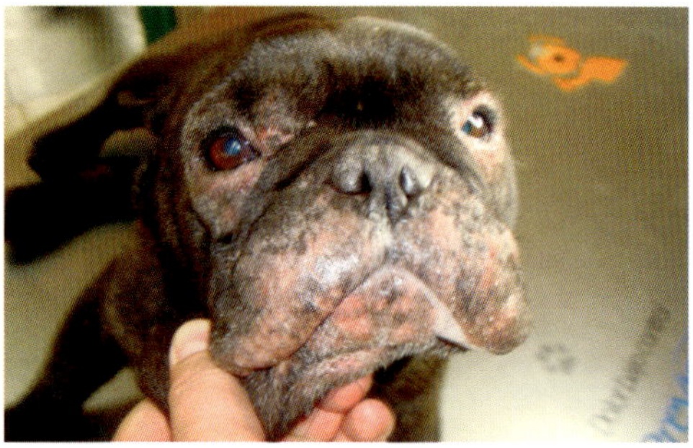

Figure 5. Deep facial pyoderma in an atopic dog.

CATS

COMMON CLINICAL SIGNS

- Self-induced alopecia.
- Miliary dermatitis.
- Head and neck dermatitis (Fig. 6).
- Eosinophilic granuloma complex.
- Faecal impaction, vomiting and constipation.

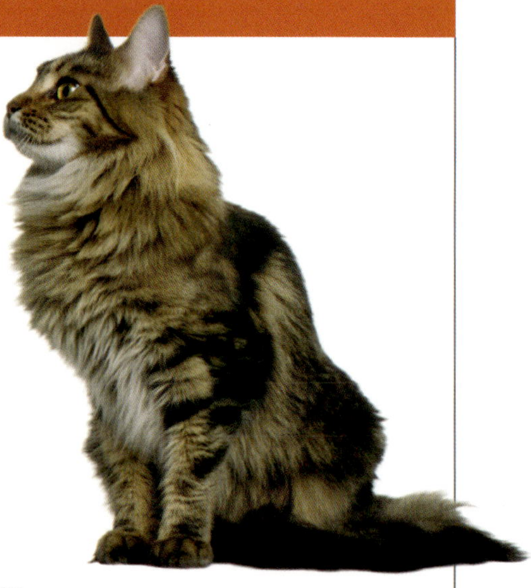

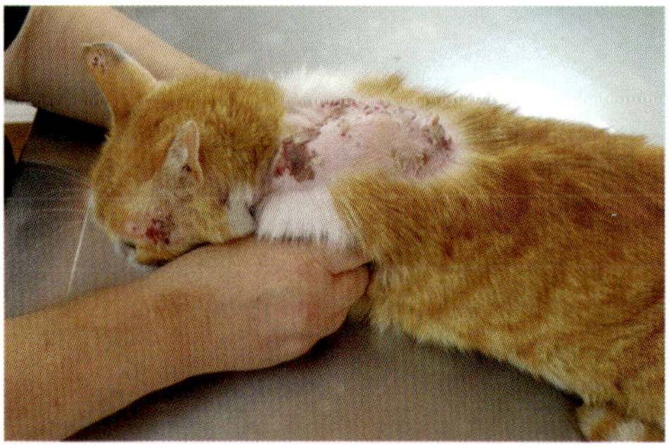

Figure 6. Cat with severe dermatitis in the cervical and supraocular areas.

RARE CLINICAL SIGNS

- Asthma and cough.
- Pyoderma.
- Otitis.
- Conjunctivitis.
- Gastrointestinal disorders.

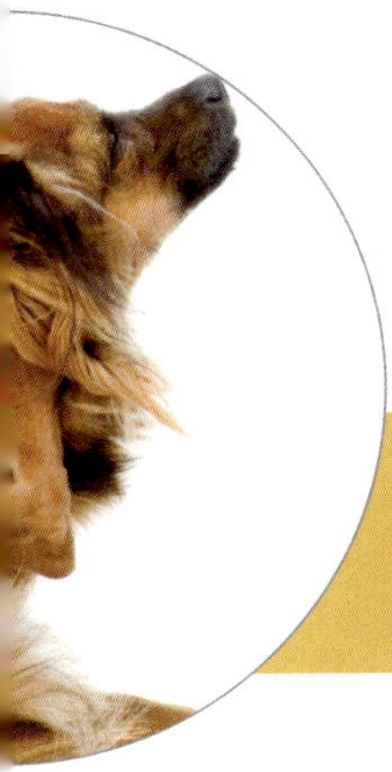

PRURITUS:
KEY SIGN IN THE ALLERGIC PATIENT

Pruritus is the most significant clinical sign of allergic dermatitis in both dogs and cats.

PRURITUS
Itch that leads to a compelling need for the animal to scratch, lick, chew, drag, roll, or shake itself. It is a complex neurodermatological reaction.

LESION–PRURITUS–SCRATCHING CYCLE

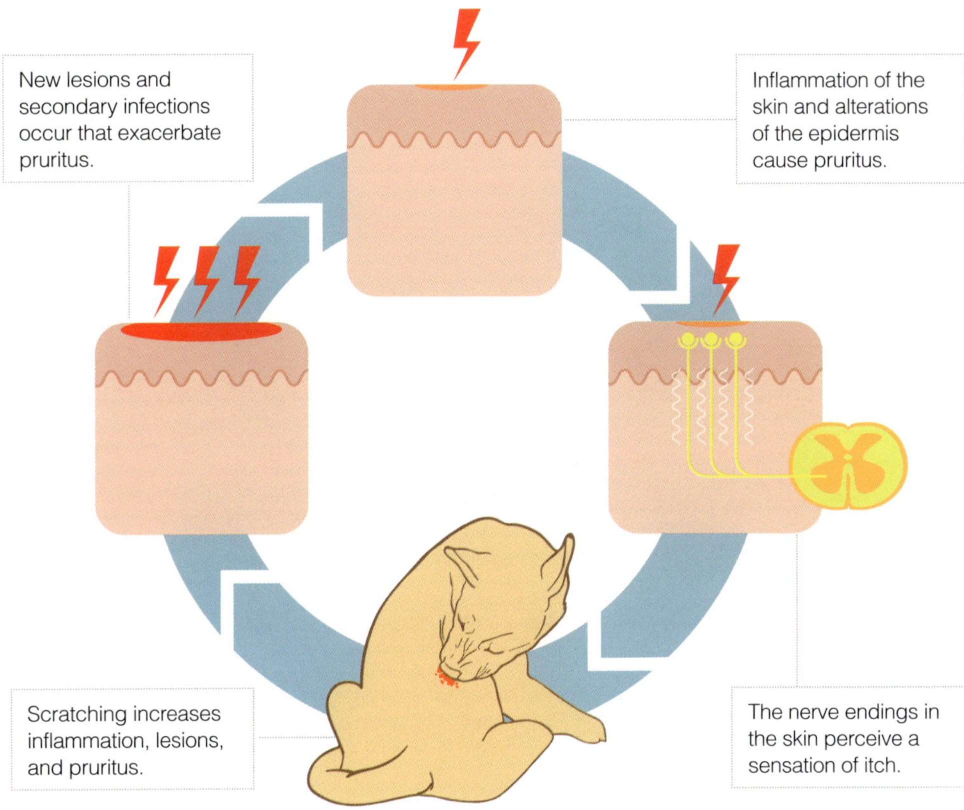

One of the interleukins that plays a leading role in pruritus in the dog, IL-31, was recently discovered.
In the cat, the process is currently not understood in as much detail.

The behavioural manifestations of pruritus vary by species.

DOGS

- It is much more obvious and self-mutilating (Fig. 7). The intensity and evidence of pruritus may be quantified subjectively on a visual scale from 1 to 10 (see table on page 14).
- Dogs use any means possible to relieve their pruritus:
  - Scratching with the paws.
  - Licking.
  - Chewing.
  - Dragging.
  - Shaking.

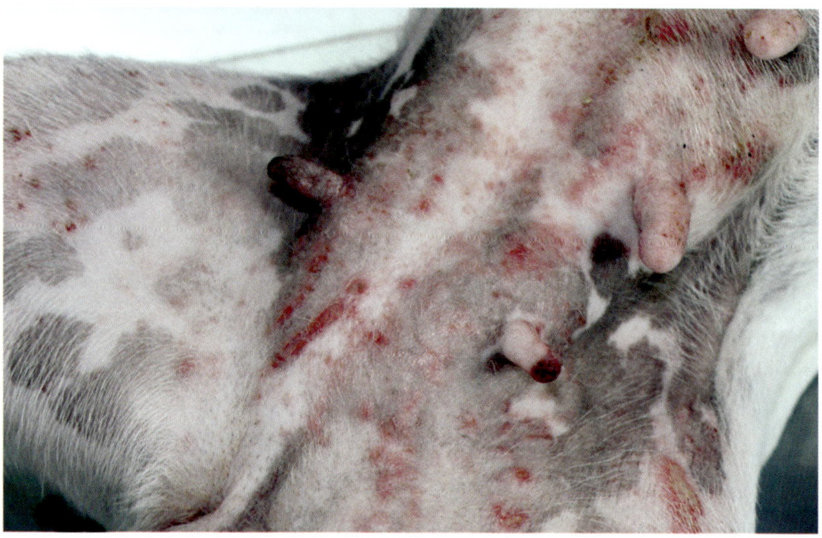

Figure 7. Classic linear excoriations on the abdomen of a dog with severe pruritus. Note the other lesions that indicate a secondary pyoderma.

CATS

- Because of their introversion, pruritus is less obvious and lesions appear less aggressive.
- Licking is very common in cats, but the papillary surface of the tongue may be abrasive (Fig. 8).
- Under some circumstances, the cat literally chews its hair out and, less often, scratches itself with its paws.
- Cats generally scratch and lick out of sight, so many owners are unable to document pruritus.

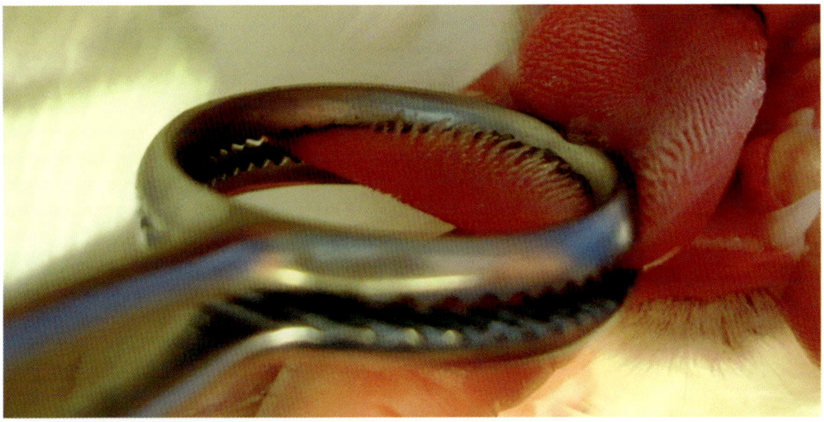

Figure 8. The papillary surface of a cat's tongue may lead to lesions during compulsive licking.

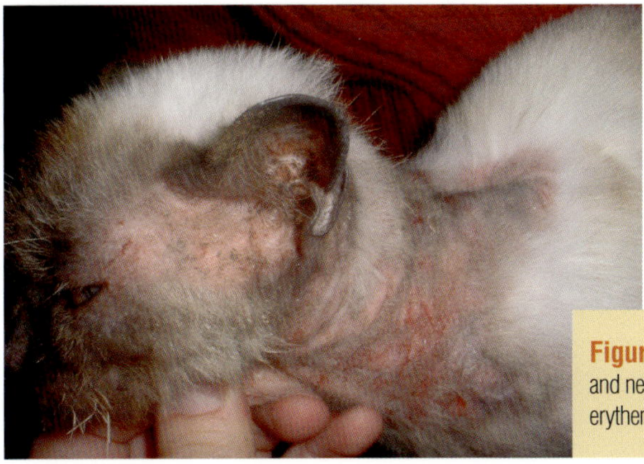

There are always special cases: for example, head and neck dermatitis with severe self-inflicted lesions (Fig. 9).

Figure 9. Excoriations in a cat with reactive head and neck dermatitis. Note the severe excoriations with erythema and scabs.

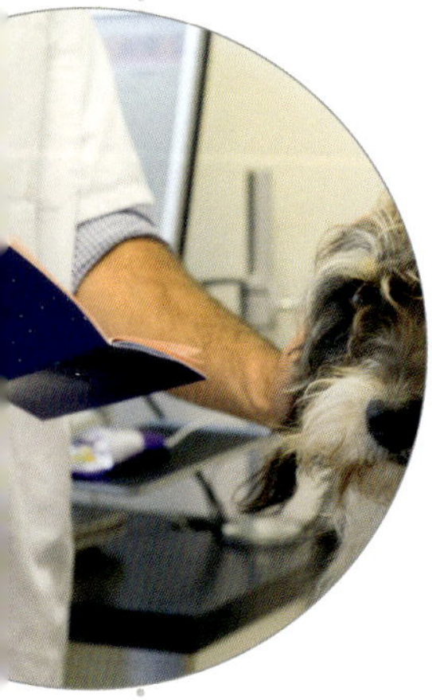

PROTOCOL
FOR CLINICAL EXAMINATION

Clinical examination serves to both confirm an allergic disease and rule out differential diagnoses.

> Be as objective as possible when examining the patient and obtain information without preconceived diagnoses.

Data from the patient's clinical record and history will inform the dermatological assessment. However, in some cases these data may bias the analysis to the exclusion of other differentials. Thus, in the case of allergic diseases, dermatological assessment is essential for making presumptive diagnoses and choosing the most suitable laboratory tests to confirm or exclude them.

THE IMPORTANCE
OF AN OVERALL HEALTH ASSESSMENT

Certain skin diseases may be caused by systemic disorders, and certain skin abnormalities may alter a patient's general health. It is therefore very important to exhaustively review the patient's case without overlooking any systemic health parameters:

- Body condition.
- Mucous membranes.
- Temperature.
- Cardiac and respiratory auscultation.
- Lymph nodes.
- Abdominal palpation.
- Status of palpable genital organs.

ALLERGY

Inappropriate or exaggerated immune response to allergens the animal inhales, ingests or comes into contact with, together with a deficiency in skin structure.

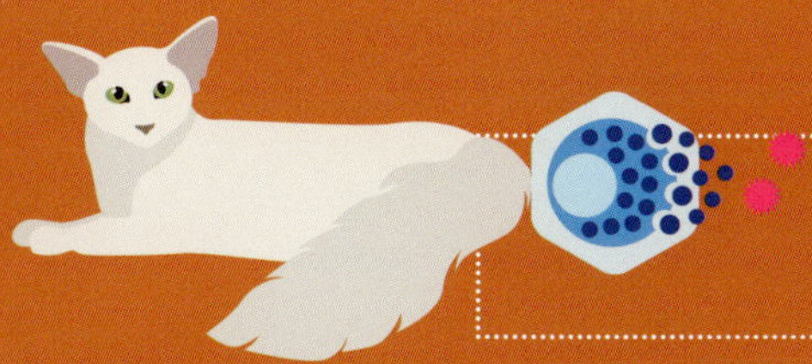

ALLERGENS

Antigens that trigger immediate or type I hypersensitivity reactions.

FOOD ALLERGY

Inappropriate or exaggerated immune response to an ingested food or ingredient.

MOST COMMON FOOD ALLERGENS

Beef, chicken, pork, lamb, eggs, milk, white fish, soya, wheat, and corn.

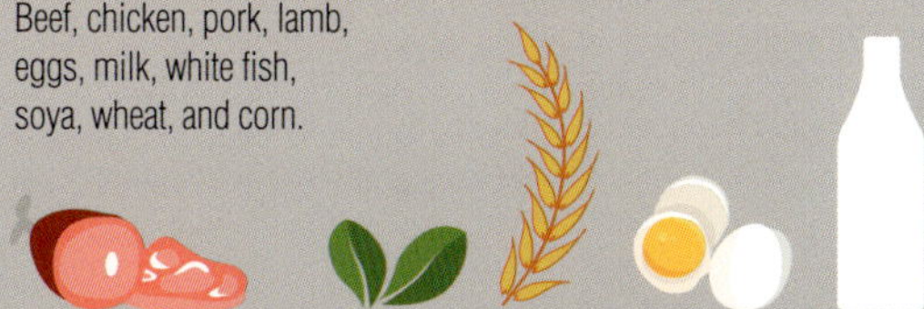

ATOPY

Allergic reaction to environmental allergens, with abnormal exposure due to skin deficiencies.

MAIN ALLERGENS RESPONSIBLE

Mites

Pollen

Mould

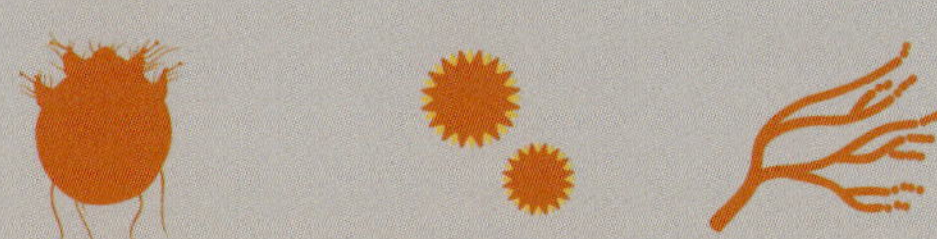

WHAT CLINICAL SIGNS DOES THE ANIMAL SHOW?

Scratching

Chewing

Excessive licking

Skin erythema

Gastrointestinal disorders

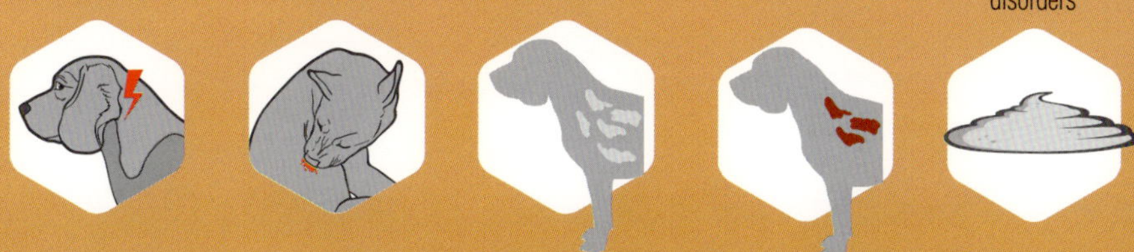

WHERE TO FOCUS?

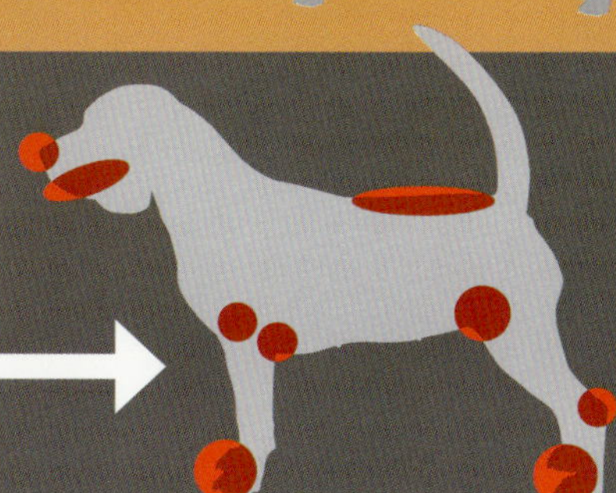

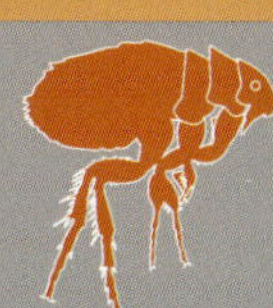

Flea allergy dermatitis (FAD) is also considered an allergic disease.

The next section describes skin diseases related to systemic allergies and abnormalities.
Body condition may be abnormal in allergic animals. Some treatments favour weight gain. However, weight loss is more likely with severe pruritus.

General and dermatological examination of the mucous membranes is very important, because pyoderma and autoimmune diseases often manifest at the mucocutaneous junctions. The mucosa itself may have ulcers, and gingivitis may occur in animals with significant pruritus. Plaque and hairs stuck between the teeth are characteristic of an animal that chews itself. As with other parts of the body, systemic diseases may also alter the colour of the mucosae (Fig. 10).

Some cats may suffer from papillitis of the tongue and even linear erosions of the hard palate from compulsive licking.

The patient's body temperature may increase and cause febrile syndromes, for example, in cases of deep pyoderma.

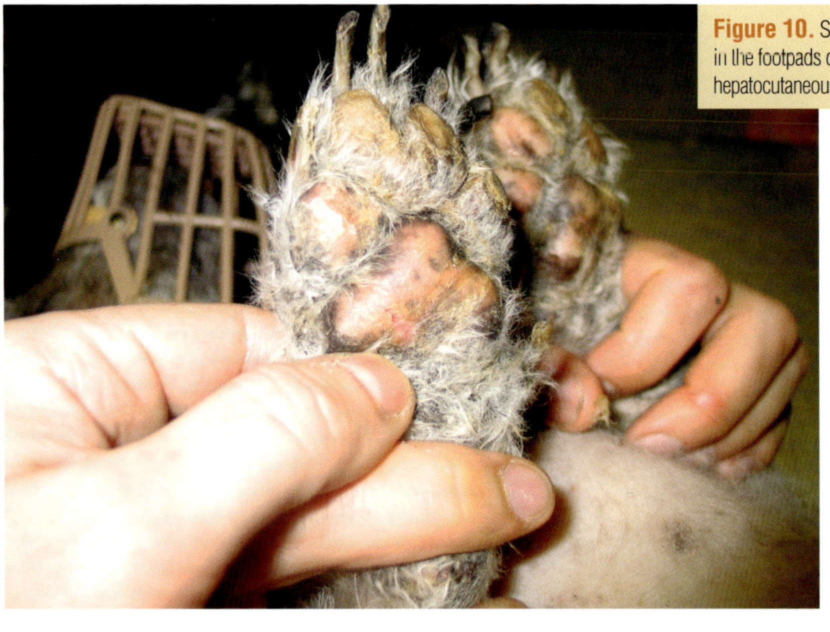

Figure 10. Significant icterus in the footpads of a dog with hepatocutaneous syndrome.

In cardiopulmonary auscultation, it is important to verify regular rhythm and heart sounds in order to rule out systemic diseases such as hypothyroidism, which can indirectly affect the skin and lead to pyoderma that causes pruritus.

Lymph nodes and sentinel lymph nodes in specific areas, if inflamed, can suggest local cutaneous infections or inflammation. Differentiate between localised and generalised lymphadenopathy.

Abdominal palpitation is very important to recognise abnormalities in abdominal organs and intestinal inflammation or pain that may be related to gastrointestinal and cutaneous diseases such as AFRs.

Regarding the genital organs, always carefully palpate the testicles and mammary glands for masses that can alter the individual's general or dermatological health (Fig. 11).

Figure 11. Testicular asymmetry. Dog with testicular sertolinoma and dermatitis.

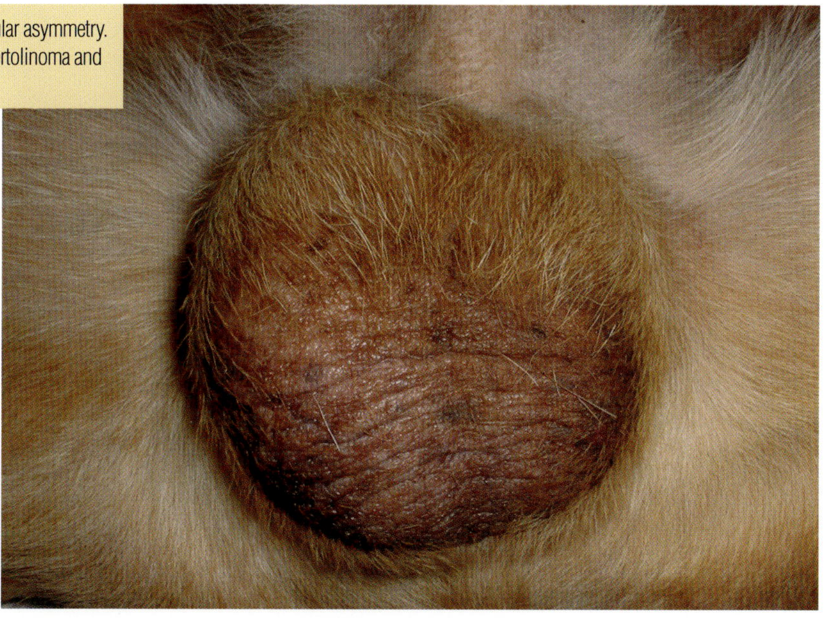

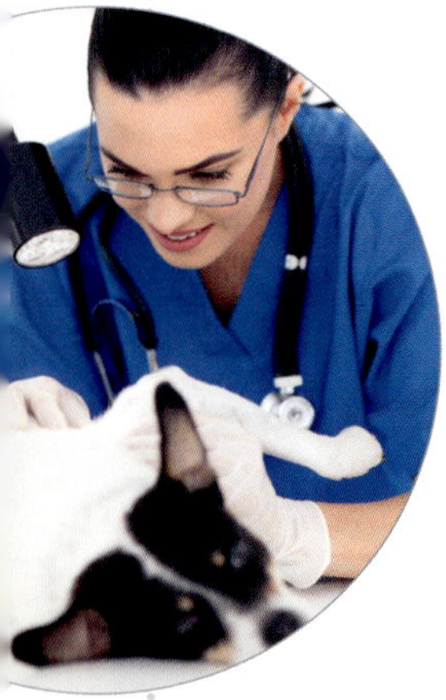

DERMATOLOGICAL
ASSESSMENT

Once the patient has been systemically examined, the skin should be systematically evaluated.

The "macro to micro" technique is highly recommended: start by generally evaluating the patient, gradually focusing on specific regions and areas, and finally honing in on particular lesions, using the dermatoscope if appropriate. The clearest example of allergy is a patient with foci of pruritus and pyoderma. The body is examined to identify affected areas and changes in hair and skin colour, alopecia, and lesions such as excoriations, erythema, papules, pustules and scabs.

Reddish fur staining, produced by oxidation of saliva, indicates where the animal has been licking or chewing.

Alopecia patterns reveal whether lesions are global, disseminated, localised or regional. Excoriations indicate the localisation and intensity of pruritus. Papules reveal release of histamine by mast cells; pustules, the possible presence of bacteria; and scabs, dried secretions such as pus or blood after exposure to the environment. Erythema is an indication of inflamed skin and may indicate allergic contact dermatitis (Fig. 12).

Figure 12. Severe erythroderma in a dog with anaphylaxis.

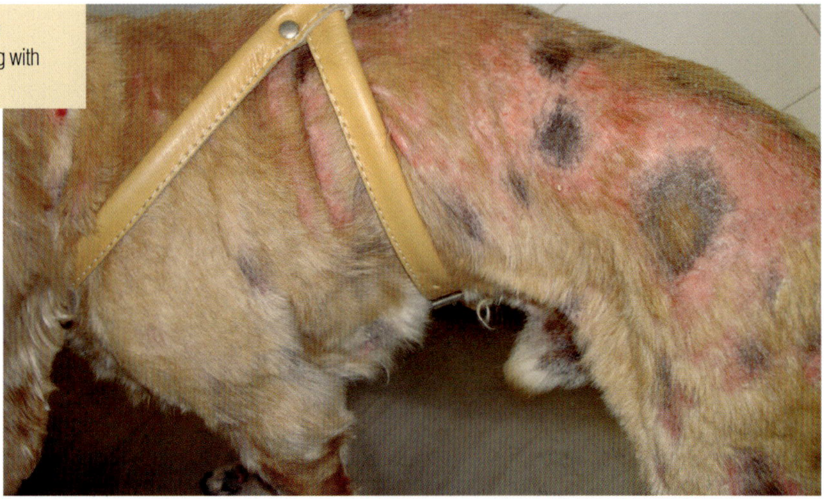

DERMATOSCOPY

This is an entirely noninvasive technique that uses a magnifying glass to observe whether lesions are follicular or extra-follicular. In some cases, it also can reveal different colour shades in the scabs, which can range from red due to blood to yellowish from pus.

THE ALLERGIC DOG: GROSS PATTERNS

Different gross patterns can indicate skin alterations due to allergy in the dog.

> Gross patterns are combinations of primary and secondary skin lesions that arise as a result of different dermatological conditions.

In allergic dogs, the most common patterns that manifest either singly or in combination are:

- Focal, multifocal, regional, generalised, diffuse, or symmetric alopecia (Fig. 13). At times, it is accompanied by fur staining from saliva. This may be self-induced by pruritus or result from folliculitis due to secondary infections.
- Erosive–ulcerative. At times it is accompanied by excoriations that indicate pruritus.
- Combined exfoliative–desquamative–seborrhoeic. Often accompanied by overgrowth of yeasts and/or bacteria.
- Papular–pustular–crusted. Highly consistent with skin infections.
- Pigmentary changes. In general, hyperpigmentation results from chronic inflammation, and hypopigmentation, mainly at the mucocutaneous junctions, is the consequence of pyoderma (Fig. 14).

Figure 13 **TYPES OF ALOPECIA**

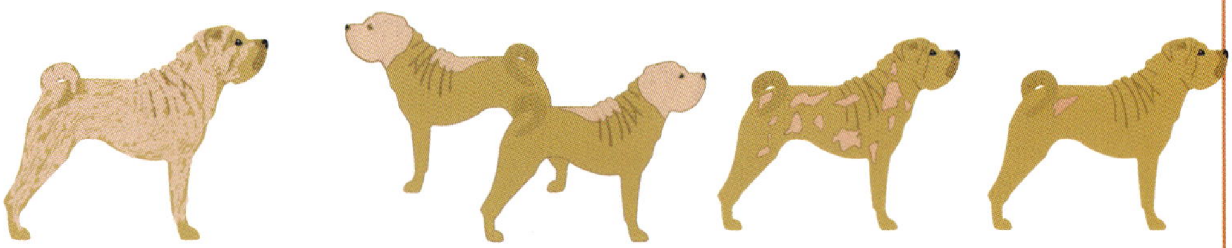

Generalised partial | Bilateral or symmetrical | Generalised multifocal | Fully localised

THE ALLERGIC CAT: REACTION PATTERNS

Cats are very special patients from a dermatological and allergic point of view. This species has very highly-developed grooming practices, which are greatly influenced by different factors.

Pruritus is a significant manifestation of allergic disease, but owners may consider excessive self-grooming due to pruritus as normal, and cats may overgroom in hiding. It is also worth noting that cats need a dynamic and rich environment for their behavioural health.

THE FOUR REACTION PATTERNS

SELF-INDUCED ALOPECIA

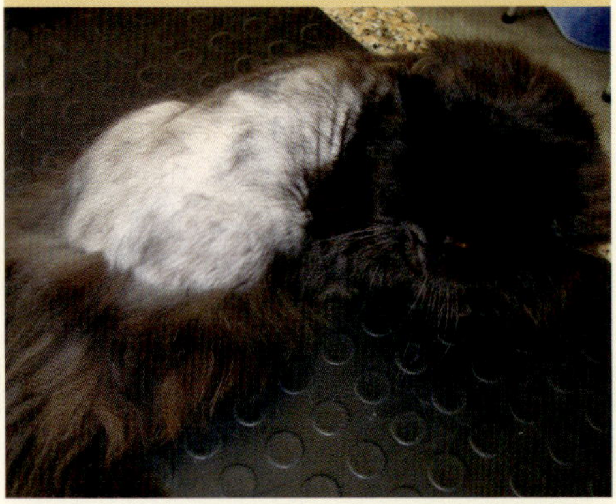

Figure 15. Self-induced alopecia. Flea allergy dermatitis in a cat.

FELINE EOSINOPHILIC GRANULOMA COMPLEX

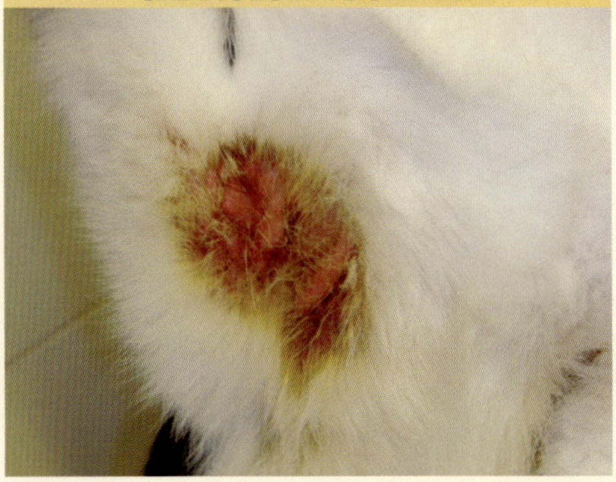

Figure 16. Axillary eosinophilic plaque in a cat with atopic-like dermatitis.

Figure 14 **SKIN DEPIGMENTATION**

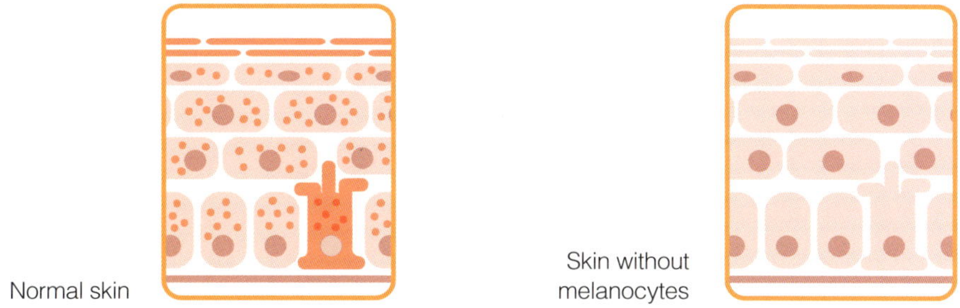

> Self-grooming due to pruritus in the cat may be confused with or differ only slightly from normal self-grooming, and it may be exacerbated by stress and lack of environmental enrichment.

The skin of cats may react to different harmful agents in four patterns that may occur singly or in combination. Note that allergies are not the sole causes of these reactions.

MILIARY DERMATITIS

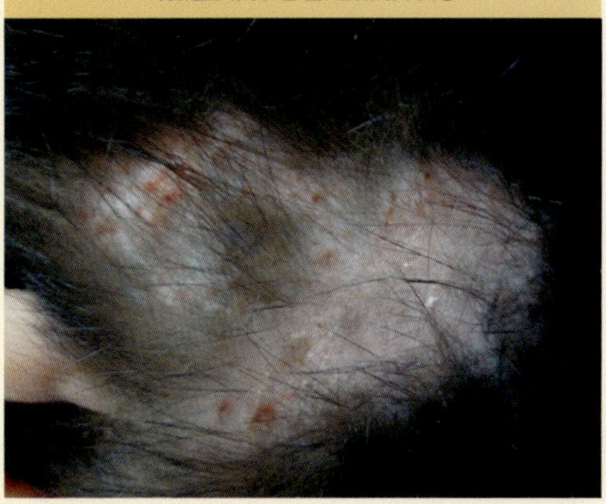

Figure 17. Miliary dermatitis pattern in an allergic cat.

HEAD AND NECK DERMATITIS

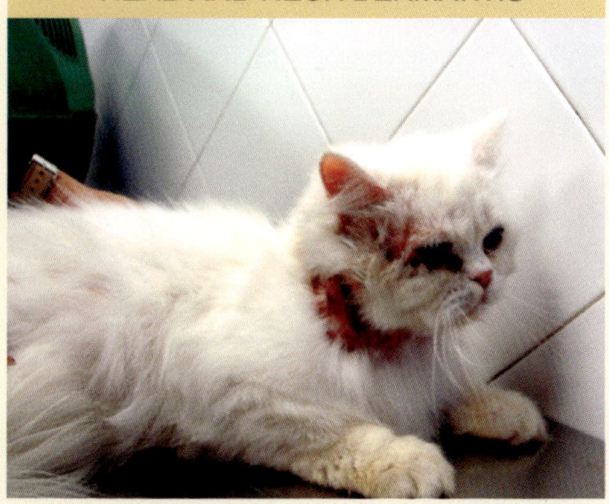

Figure 18. Head and neck dermatitis pattern in a cat with AFR.

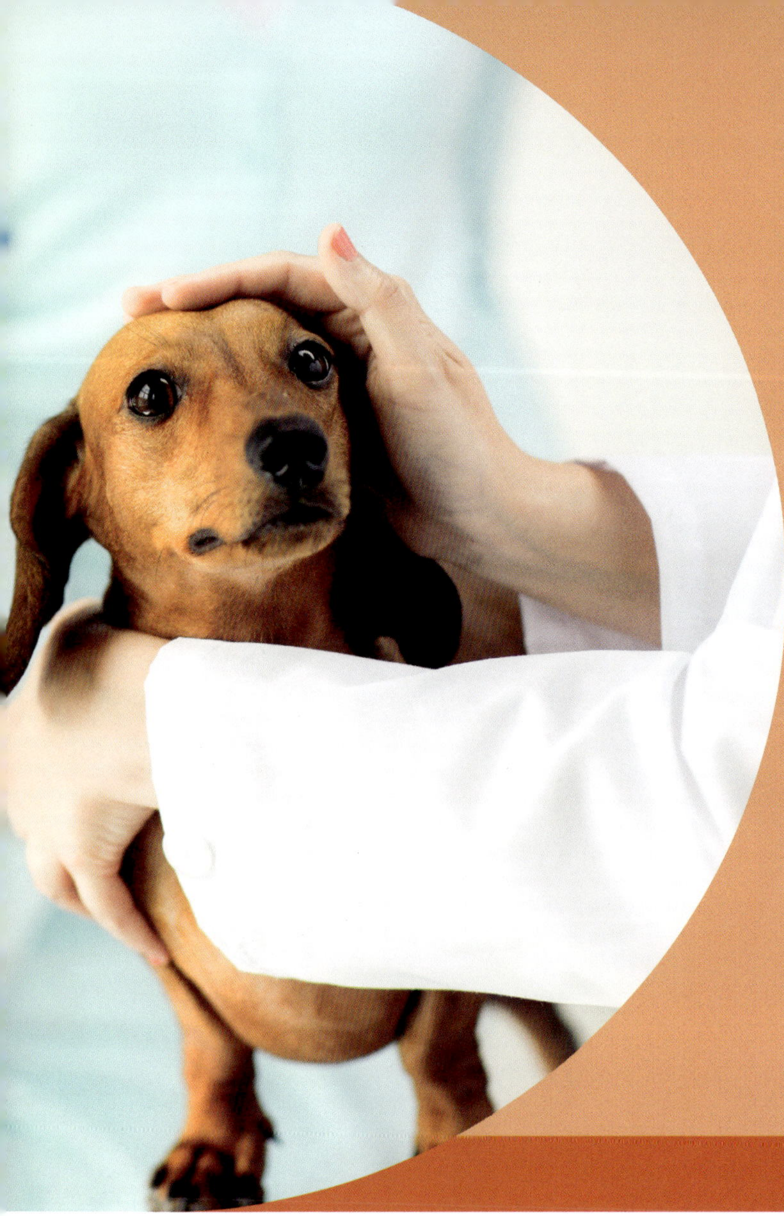

2

DIAGNOSTIC PROTOCOLS

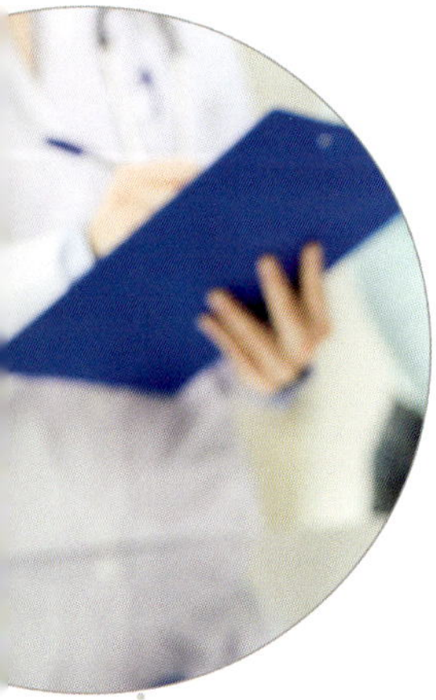

HOW TO MAKE
PRESUMPTIVE DIAGNOSES.
DIFFERENTIAL DIAGNOSIS

This guide covers the following most common allergic diseases:

- Urticaria, angioedema.
- Canine atopic dermatitis or feline atopic-like dermatitis.
- Food allergy dermatitis.
- Flea allergy dermatitis.
- Hypersensitivity to mosquito bite.
- Hypersensitivity to insect sting. Eosinophilic forunculosis.
- Hypersensitivity to ear mites *(Otodectes cynotis)*.
- Contact dermatitis.
- Drug hypersensitivity.

Allergic animals that are genetically predisposed may have one or more of these hypersensitivities. This chapter will discuss the three most common (by far), which are: atopic dermatitis, food allergy dermatitis and flea allergy dermatitis. Clinically, these are often seen in combination and may be considered as differentials when attempting to diagnose the predominant condition.

The selection of presumptive diagnoses is very important in the dermatological protocol.

The veterinary surgeon must therefore combine all the data from the history together with the findings of the full examination and select the most likely diagnoses.

The general appearance of the patient, combined with the distribution of lesions, their likely origin, and the information the owner provides on the animal's behaviour will steer the clinician towards possible diagnoses.

The history is as important as the owner's comments about the intensity and localisation of the pruritus and may be essential when making a diagnosis (Table 1).

IMPORTANCE OF THE HISTORY

Cause	Pruritus			
	Intensity	Type	Region	Frequency
Scabies/*Notoedres*	High	Skin scrape	Elbows, ears, legs, anus	High
Presence of fleas	Low–medium	Episodes; scratching, chewing	Ventral abdomen and thighs. Radius, carpus, tibia, tarsus	Low–medium
Other parasites	Low, medium, or high, depending on infestation	Scratching, chewing	Highly variable	Low–medium
FAD	High	Chewing, scratching	Dorsal, lumbar, tail	High
CAD/feline hypersensitivity	High	Scratching, chewing, licking, dragging, shaking	Face and paws Thighs, radius, carpus, tibia, tarsus, except lesions	High
Infection and xerosis secondary to endocrine diseases/seborrhoea	Low–medium	Licking–chewing	Highly variable	Low–medium
Immune-mediated/ systemic diseases	Highly variable, medium–high depending on infection	Scratching, licking	Generalised. Nose, footpads, ears	Medium
Neoplastic: SCC, lymphoma, NME; paraneoplastic	Highly variable, medium	Scratching, licking	Extensive. Depends on areas affected. Mucocutaneous	Medium
Behavioural	Highly variable	Licking, chewing	Areas affected	Medium–high
Viral, neurogenic	Medium–high	Licking, chewing, self-mutilation	Limbs, other regions	High

FAD: flea-allergy dermatitis, cad: canine atopic dermatitis, SCC: squamous cell carcinoma, NME: necrolytic migratory erythema.

Table 1. Comparison between the types and intensities of pruritus, with localisation and frequency.

> A good diagnostic approach is analysing the individual as a whole and being as specific as possible.

Understanding the formation of lesions and their molecular mechanism reveals their origin and highlights the most likely disease.

For example, if a dog presents with papules and pustules in the axillae and groin along with pruritus and licking, these lesions were likely caused by scratching as a sign of pruritus in areas commonly affected in allergic animals. The next step is to ask why these pustules occurred and how they formed. The most likely explanation is bacterial dissemination from licking and scratching with the paws. This can be confirmed by examining the content of the pustules for granulocytes and bacteria. These lesions fuel the pruritus, yielding a vicious cycle that must be treated. The common thread of this problem in allergic patients is insufficient control of the microbiota because of abnormalities in the skin's structure and microbicidal substances.

The table below shows the most common causes of pruritus (the most significant clinical sign) by age of onset (Table 2):

PRURITUS. MOST LIKELY CAUSES BY AGE				
Young (<1 year)		1–5 years	>5 years	
≤5 months	>6 months		5–8 years	>8 years
➤ Hypersensitivity due to intestinal parasites ➤ External parasites ➤ Neurogenic	➤ CAD/AFR ➤ Infection/CAD/AFR ➤ External parasites ➤ Neurogenic	➤ CAD/ARF ➤ Infection/CAD/ARF ➤ External parasites ➤ Neurogenic ➤ Drug reaction ➤ Behavioural	➤ Endocrine disease/Infection ➤ CAD/AFR /Infection ➤ Parasites ➤ Autoimmune ➤ Neurogenic ➤ Drug reaction ➤ Behavioural	➤ Neoplastic ➤ CAD/ARF/Infection ➤ External parasites ➤ Autoimmune ➤ Neurogenic ➤ Drug reaction ➤ Behavioural/referred pain ➤ Endocrine disease

Table 2. Most likely causes of pruritus by age. CAD: canine atopic dermatitis, AFR: adverse food reaction.

Given that pruritus is a common sign of various diseases, a diagram of differential diagnoses and the most commonly used laboratory tests (Fig. 1) is shown below:

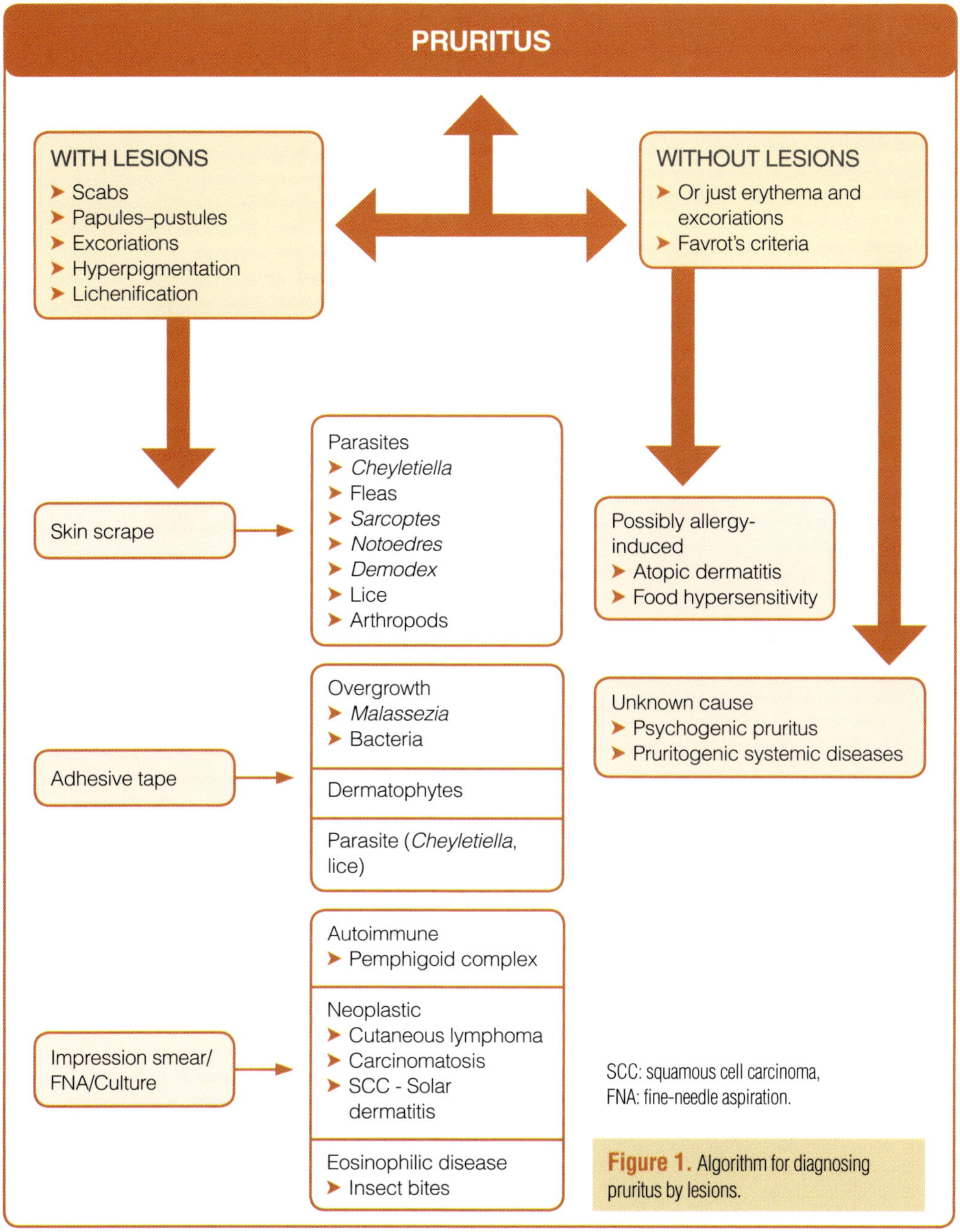

SCC: squamous cell carcinoma, FNA: fine-needle aspiration.

Figure 1. Algorithm for diagnosing pruritus by lesions.

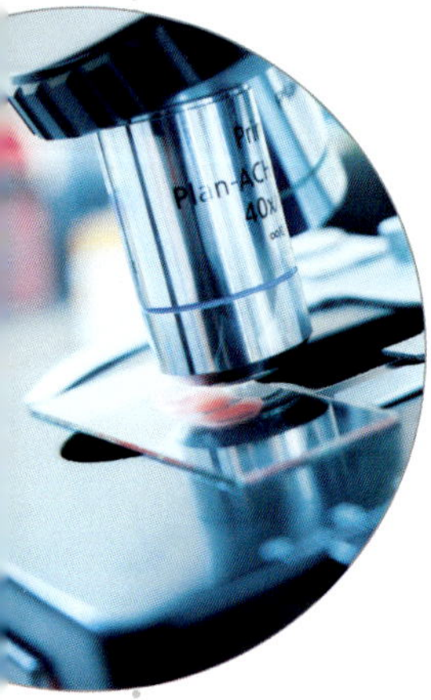

LABORATORY TESTS

Once a list of presumptive diagnoses has been developed in order from most to least likely, the most highly indicated laboratory test should be selected to confirm or rule out differential diagnoses in order of likelihood. At this stage of the protocol, the veterinary clinician's experience and expertise play an important role in selecting the best follow-up method, starting with the cheapest and simplest.

Obviously, differential diagnoses in this text relate to allergies.

USE OF A FINE COMB OR BRUSH

In the event of a possible allergy, the first differential diagnosis is the presence of fleas is flea allergy. Fleas can exacerbate or cause allergic signs, so fleas must be absent to measure the actual extent of any allergic signs.

The ideal procedure is wetting the patient's fur against the grain with a strong liquid insecticide five minutes before brushing or combing. Next, brushing is performed and the debris is collected on an absorbent white paper that will show fleas and/or flea faeces. These manifest as small dots that dissolve and stain the paper reddish-brown.

A spray suitable for both cats and dogs, such as fipronil, is usually used.

This method serves to differentiate the causes of parasitic pruritus:

- Fleas.
- Lice.
- *Cheyletiella* (Fig. 2).
- Mites.

> **TIP**
>
> Apply the spray to the dorsal area and look for fleas escaping to the ventral area of the animal's body, which is usually highly visible due to being hairless.

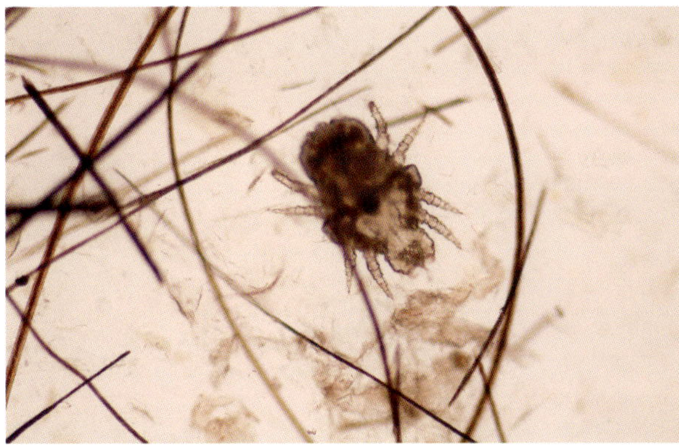

Figure 2. *Cheyletiella* observed by brushing.

ADHESIVE TAPE

This is the most common additional method used in allergic patients, mainly dogs. A good transparent adhesive tape with strong adhesive power can be used to collect samples from different areas of the body, stain them, and examine for microbial overgrowth, and in some cases, the presence of neutrophils (which suggest anomalies at a deeper level). It is best to apply tape to hairless areas with erythema and seborrhoea or with lichenification and hyperpigmentation.

The observation of bacteria and/or yeast, together with mostly keratinised epithelial cells, confirms microbial overgrowth, which appears grossly as skin areas with alopecia, seborrhoea and hyperpigmentation, or erythema. These skin disorders are characteristic of atopic animals who may have deficiencies either in their skin's structure or its production of bacteriostatic or mycostatic substances, such as certain fatty acids and peptides.

There is a very important differential diagnosis for allergy: cheyletiellosis. In this case, the use of adhesive tape is ideal.

This method shows:

- Microbial overgrowth (Fig. 3).
- Superficial parasites.
- Superficial cells.

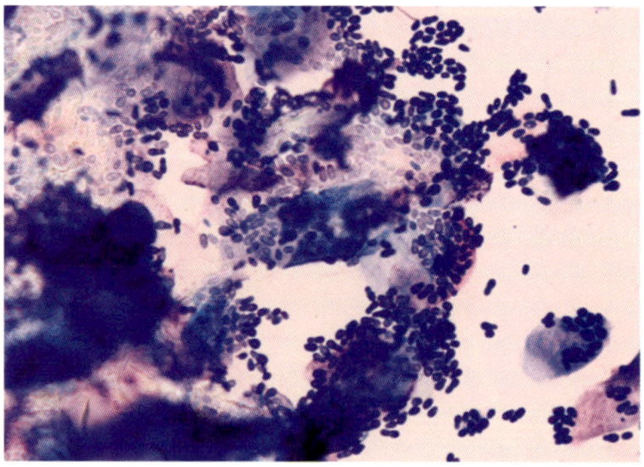

Figure 3. *Malassezia* overgrowth observed with adhesive tape.

IMPRESSION
CYTOLOGY

For allergies, this procedure is very similar to that of adhesive tape: press the glass slide onto an affected area. The advantage is better staining of the sample on the slide; the disadvantage is that it is not possible to obtain impressions of irregular surfaces, such as the interdigital spaces.

> With this method, samples of deeper or exudative lesions can be obtained.

Diff quik staining is ideal for both methods mentioned above, although it works better on the glass slide. The adhesive tape usually only uses the blue component of the panoptic or methylene blue; the red stain can also be used, but never the fixator, as this will remove the adhesive material from the tape.

This additional method shows:

- Bacterial overgrowth (Fig. 4).
- Yeast overgrowth.
- Inflammatory cells suggesting abnormalities at a deeper level.
- Neoplastic cytology.

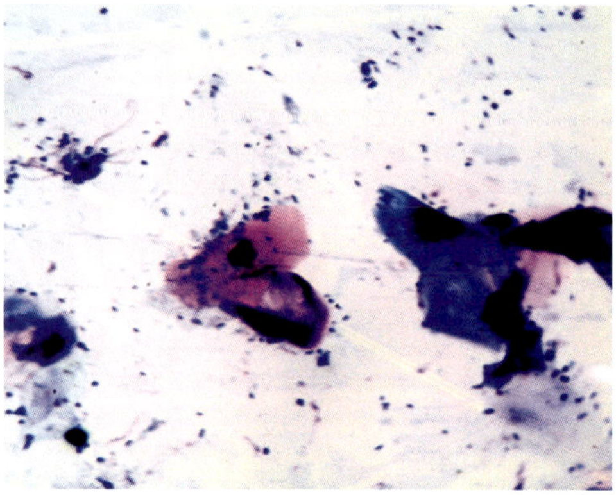

Figure 4. Bacterial overgrowth obtained by impression. Note the keratinocytes and bacteria.

SKIN SCRAPING

Skin scraping is a very common method used mainly to check for parasites that can produce or exacerbate allergic-type signs (Table 3).

Superficial and deep scraping may reveal *Sarcoptes scabiei* or *Demodex* type mites (Fig. 5).

Superficial skin scrapes may be used for cytology, especially those taken under scabs, or to search for certain kinds of *Demodex*, which are typically observed in atopic breeds such as the West Highland White Terrier or Fox Terrier (in which they can cause seborrhoeic dermatitis) and are usually found in superficial areas of the skin and in dorsal plaques.

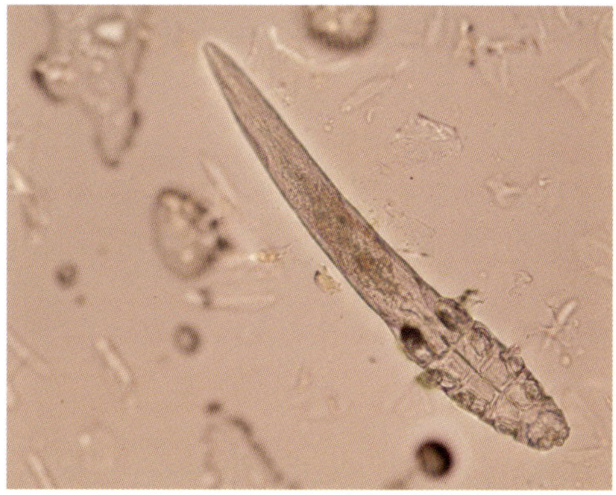

Figure 5. *Demodex injai* in a superficial skin scrape.

Superficial skin scrape
Cheyletiella *Trombicula* *Otodectes*
Medium-depth skin scrape
Sarcoptes *Notoedres*
Deep skin scrape
Demodex *Pelodera* *Straelensia cynotis* (very difficult to detect because it is very deep and encysted)

Table 3. Types of parasites and depth of scrape necessary to detect them.

TRICHOGRAPHY

This method consists of plucking a small group of hairs from a representative area with haemostats, pulling in the direction of hair growth to avoid breaking the hairs, and removing them intact from the root. The hairs should be grasped with the haemostats as close as possible to the skin.

These hairs are placed neatly on a glass slide and secured with transparent adhesive tape on top (Fig. 6).

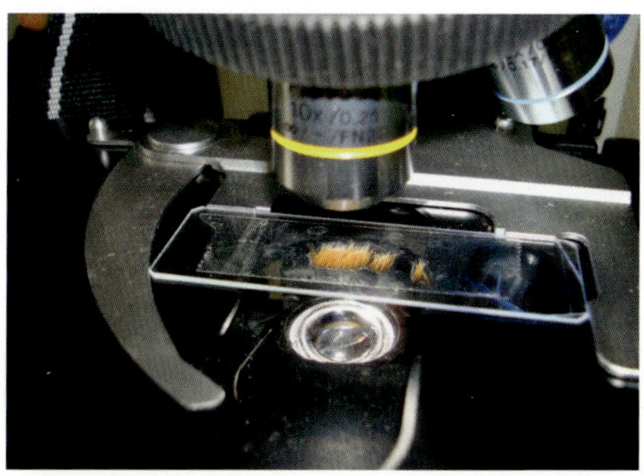

Figure 6. Placement of hairs for trichography.

The technique enables the clinician to observe the hair structure and check for parasites and/or their eggs. Certain follicular dysplasias can be accompanied by keratinisation disorders with comedones and xerosis and may be confused with an allergy because of the reactive pruritus (Fig. 7).

Trichography may reveal follicular casts that result from inflammation of the follicular wall and are characteristic of demodicosis and sebaceous adenitis.

This method helps to differentiate allergies from:

- *Demodex* (Fig. 8).
- Dysplastic hair structure
- Dermatophytosis.
- Lice and their eggs.
- *Cheyletiella* and their eggs.
- Confirm pruritus due to broken tips.

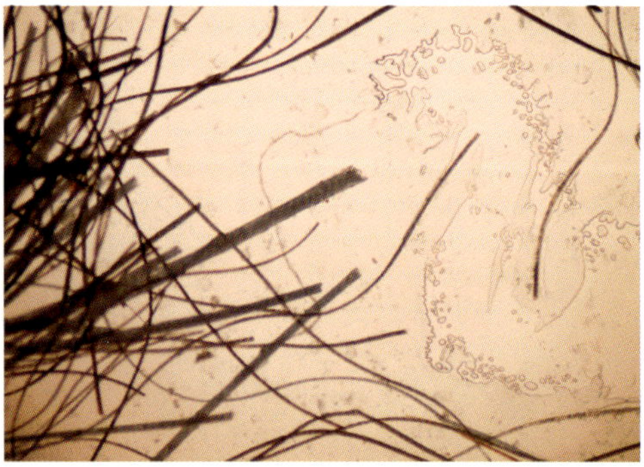

Figure 7. Trichogram from a patient with pruritus. Note the broken hairs.

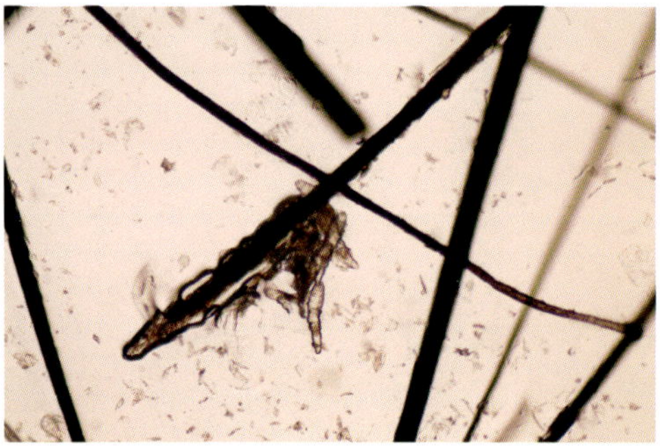

Figure 8. *Demodex* on trichography.

FINE-NEEDLE SAMPLING AND CYTOLOGY

This method is used to extract samples from nodules, tumours or papules/pustules. Different calibre needles are used based on the dimensions of the lesion or affected site, and aspiration may be used to obtain the sample. The content collected by simply introducing the needle is often sufficient.

This content should be expelled from the needle using air from a syringe. The tip of this needle can then be used to make a smear of homogeneous thickness. The smear can also be made by laying a second glass slide onto the sample and smoothly moving the slides apart. The smear on the glass slide is subsequently stained to be later dried and examined.

If the sample is lipid, heat fixation is necessary. Avoid alcohol fixation, which will extract the lipids.

In the case of cats, the eosinophilic reaction pattern must be confirmed by the existence of eosinophils in most of these lesions (Fig. 11).

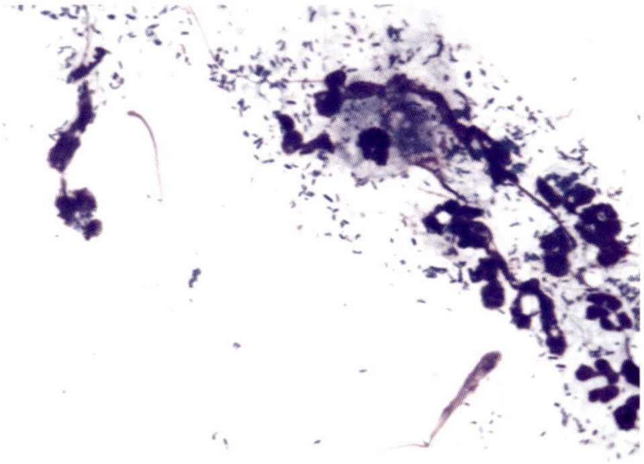

Figure 9. Cytology of deep pyoderma. Note the abundant degenerate inflammatory cells and bacilli.

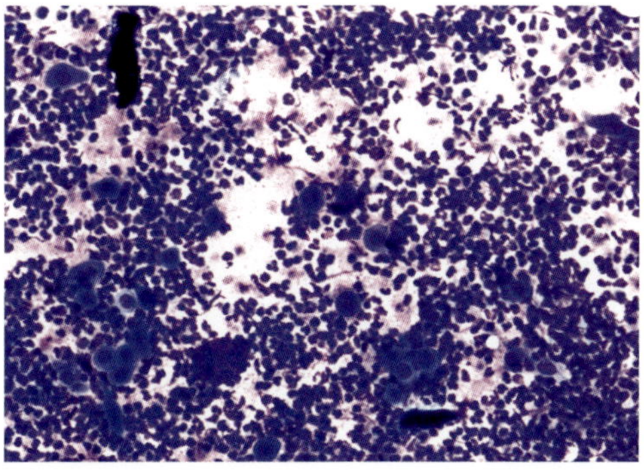

Figure 10. Cytology of a pustule in a case of pemphigus foliaceus. Note the acanthocytes and abundant neutrophils.

> This method is very useful to obtain samples from pustules to determine bacterial pathology (Fig. 9) or to differentiate from sterile causes of pruritus, as in the case of pemphigus (Fig. 10).

This method helps to differentiate allergies from:

- Pyoderma of other origin.
- Pemphigoid diseases.
- Eosinophilic diseases.
- Sterile pyogranuloma (Fig. 12).
- Neoplasms.

The aim of this book is not to cover a topic as broad and interesting as cytology but to suggest that veterinary clinicians should strive to differentiate inflammatory cells from neoplastic cells.

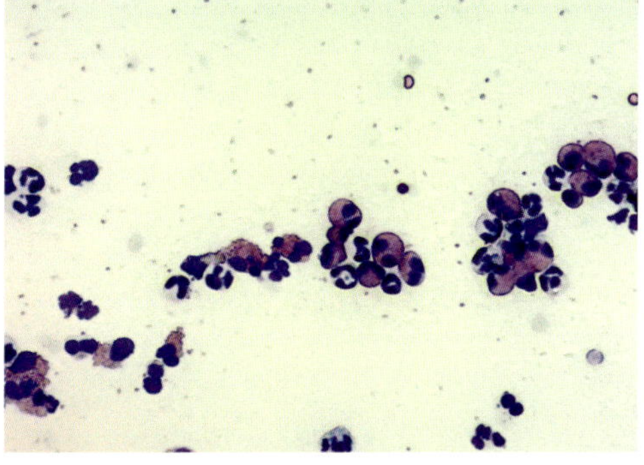

Figure 11. Cytology of an eosinophilic granuloma in a cat.

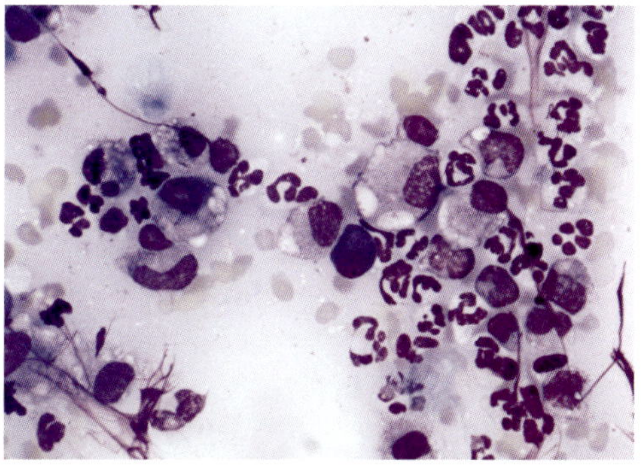

Figure 12. Cytology of a pyogranuloma. Note the activated macrophages and pyknotic neutrophils.

This method can also be used to determine whether inflammation is pyogenic (Fig. 13), granulomatous or pyogranulomatous. The kind of micro-organism involved, including yeast, cocci and bacilli, can also be studied. Finally, if a neoplasm is detected, which clinicians can learn to do, the cellular lineage can be identified as round, epithelial or mesenchymal (Figs. 14–16).

Another method to obtain a superficial sample for cytology is the swab (Fig. 17). It is very important to wet the swab with sterile saline and then obtain the sample. The sample is then transferred onto the slide for fixation and staining by rolling the swab across the slide.

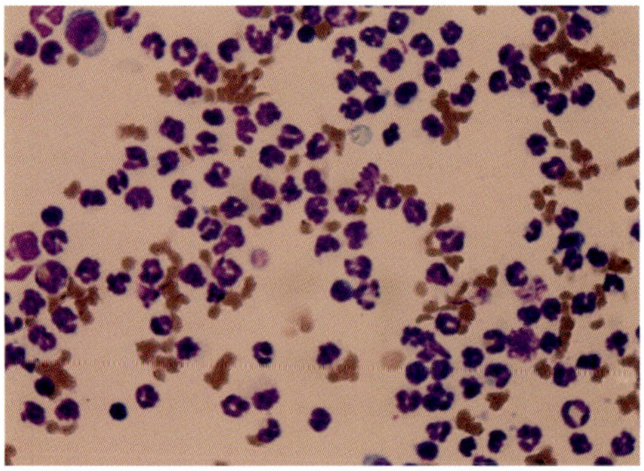

Figure 13. Pyogenic inflammation.

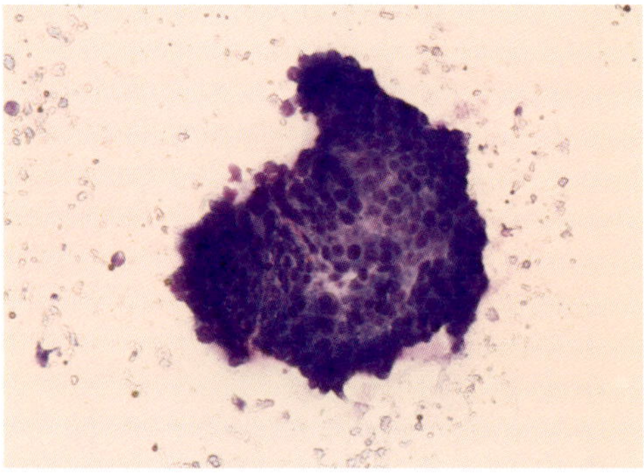

Figure 14. Epithelial lineage in cells in a cluster. Note the congruence of the cell walls.

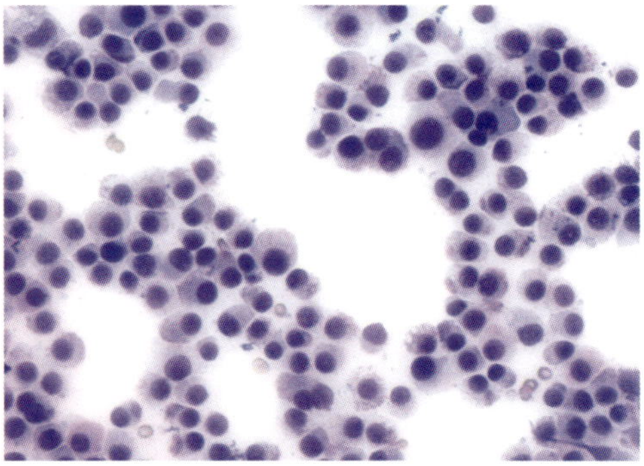

Figure 15. Round lineage cells; they are abundant and distinct.

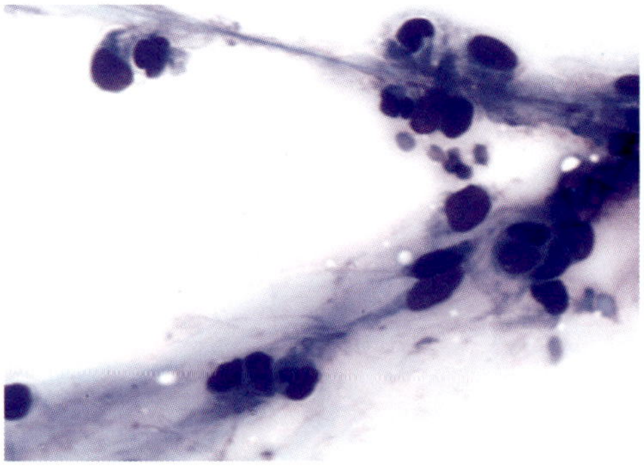

Figure 16. Mesenchymal lineage cells. They are usually few in number if they are benign.

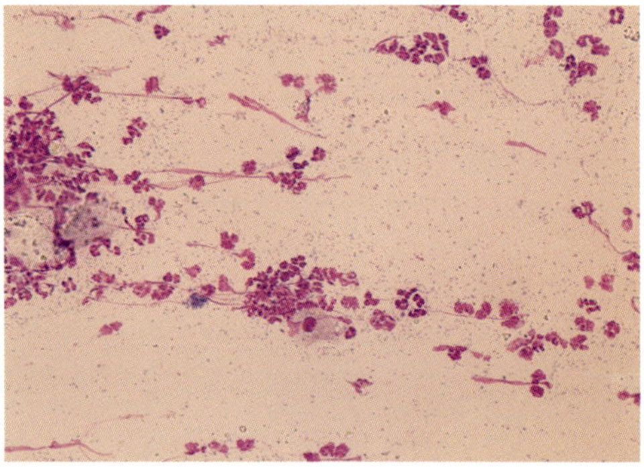

Figure 17. Swab cytology from a patient with otitis. Note the neutrophils, macrophages, cocci, and bacilli.

WOOD'S LAMP

This method is very useful for screening for dermatophytes. A high percentage of *Microsporum canis* can yield a positive test, which detects fluorescence emitted by pteridine, a fungal metabolite. This greenish-blue fluorescence can be seen in areas where hairs emerge from the skin – that is, close to the root (Fig. 18). Avoid confusion with fluorescence produced by illumination of scabs or some ointments or antiseptics.

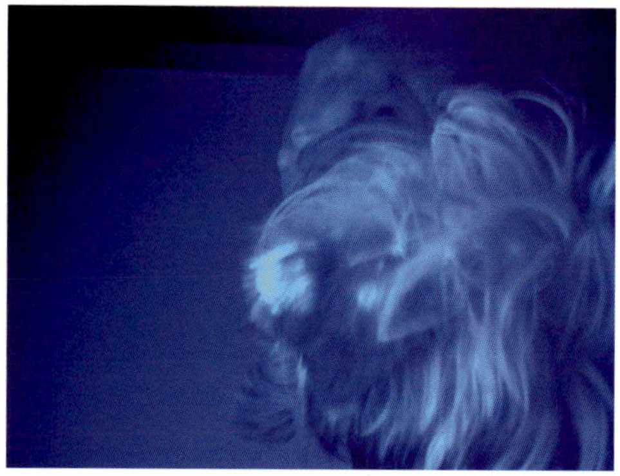

Figure 18. Positive fluorescence of hairs under Wood's lamp.

In many cases of dermatophytosis in the Yorkshire Terrier breed, highly pruritic furuncular lesions can occur, which differentiates these from allergy.

This method must be performed in a dark room to see proper light contrast.

CULTURES AND ANTIBIOTIC SENSITIVITY TESTS

Veterinary practices generally send samples for culture and antibiotic sensitivity tests to laboratories specialised in these methods.

In the case of dermatophytes, in-house cultures are available with the dye phenol red as an indicator of development of colonies. If these colonies are suspicious in colour and appearance, the veterinary surgeon should examine them for macroconidia (Fig. 19).

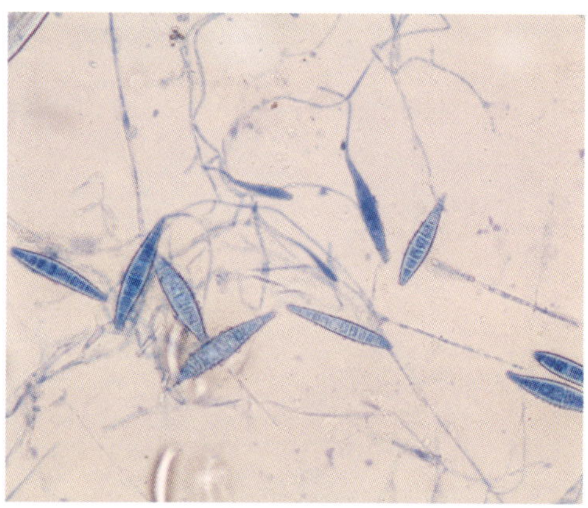

Figure 19. Macroconidia from *Microsporum canis.*

Bacterial culture and antibiotic sensitivity tests are much more difficult to perform and require special equipment and training. The recent evolution of methicillin-resistant strains and other multidrug-resistant bacteria makes this process ever more important, and now it is nearly essential.

The incidence of pyoderma and otitis refractory to treatment has prompted the use of these laboratory tests to identify the most suitable antibiotics.

> Recurrent pyoderma is a common secondary sign in many allergic patients, so it is important to verify bacterial sensitivity and its classification.

Conquering this kind of "superbacteria" often requires the prudent use of antibiotics and topical treatments, mainly antiseptics.

Culture and antibiotic sensitivity are essential in these cases:
- Presence of bacilli.
- Recurrent pyoderma or bacterial otitis.
- Deep pyoderma.

The key to obtaining a representative sample is going to the actual source of the problem. In the case of deep or recurrent pyoderma, the best sampling method consists of removing part of a biopsy sample and placing it in saline solution for culture. It is important to remove the superficial part of this tissue to avoid contamination. In cases of otitis, samples from the middle ear, separate samples from the vertical and horizontal ear canals, and separate samples from each ear are fundamental.

DIAGNOSTIC CRITERIA
OF ALLERGIES

Atopic dermatitis/adverse food reaction is a disease that generally does not require laboratory tests for diagnosis.

The patient's clinical condition and certain established tools enable diagnosis with a high degree of certainty.

DOGS*

Favrot's diagnostic criteria for atopic dermatitis

1. Onset of signs before 3 years of age.
2. Onset of pruritus prior to lesions.
3. Good response to corticosteroid treatments and possibly oclacitinib.
4. Mainly indoor animal.
5. Forelimbs affected.
6. Ears affected.
7. Ear margins free of lesions.
8. Dorsolumbar region free of lesions.

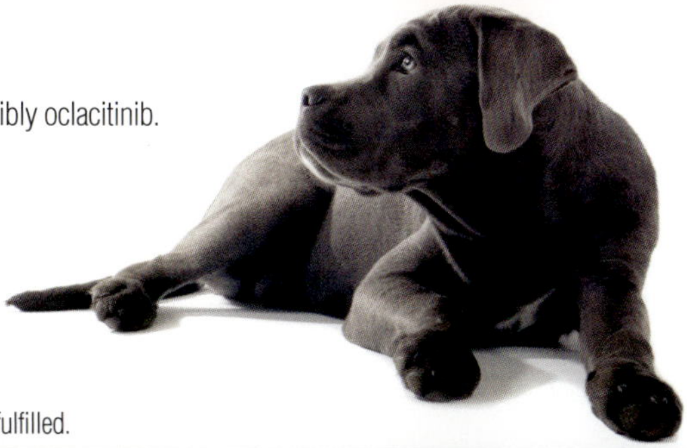

*Sensitivity and specificity approximately 80% if five criteria are fulfilled.

CATS*

Favrot's diagnostic criteria for atopic-like dermatitis

1. Presence of pruritus since onset.
2. Presence of at least two of the following clinical signs:
   - Symmetrical alopecia.
   - Crusted papular dermatitis or miliary dermatitis.
   - Plaque or nodular dermatitis (lesions of the feline eosinophilic granuloma complex).
   - Erosions or ulcers in the cervical and facial region.
3. At least two locations affected.
4. Miliary dermatitis as the predominant pattern.
5. Eosinophilic dermatitis, symmetrical alopecia, or erosions or ulcers in the cervical region, head, lips, or ears.
6. Nonsymmetrical alopecia in the dorsocaudal region, tail, or hindlimbs.
7. Symmetrical alopecia on the abdomen.
8. Absence of erosions or ulcers on the forelimbs.
9. Absence of lesions in the axillary and sternal regions.
10. Absence of nodules or tumours.

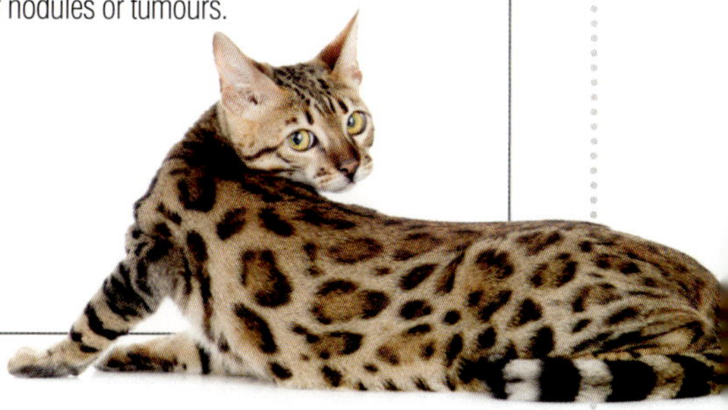

*Sensitivity 90 % and specificity approximately 83 % if six criteria are met.

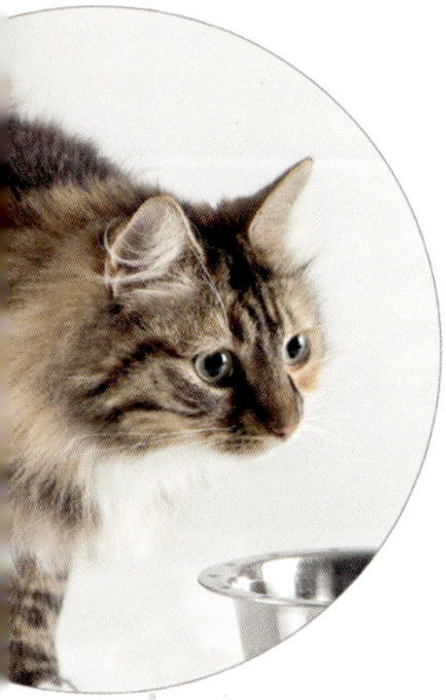

SEARCH FOR AND CONFIRMATION
OF ALLERGENS

Allergen testing in allergic diseases can be performed in cats and dogs; the purpose is to understand these allergens in an effort to avoid or minimise exposure or to develop specific immunotherapies to desensitise the patient.

Intradermal skin tests can be performed in practice using extracts of the appropriate allergens for each geographic area (Fig. 20). This is considered the gold standard to confirm possible sensitivities. However, the disadvantage is that performing this test requires a great deal of clinical training. Addition of allergen extract to the skin scrape test (Prick test) is in development, but the reference standards have not yet been determined.

Serum measurement of specific IgE can be performed in a laboratory.

Regarding food allergens, measurement of IgG and IgE specific to different foods is still not sufficient for positive diagnosis, although the negative predictive value may be useful for the design of novel ingredient diets.

Currently, the only way to diagnose or confirm the food-related origin of an allergy is to eliminate these allergens temporarily and subsequently reintroduce them as a challenge to confirm the reaction. Elimination diets involve ingredients to which the animal has not been previously exposed or commercial diets with hydrolysed proteins of a molecular size that makes them much less allergenic. These elimination diets must be maintained strictly for 8 to 10 weeks, and the challenge is subsequently performed with individual ingredients every 7–10 days.

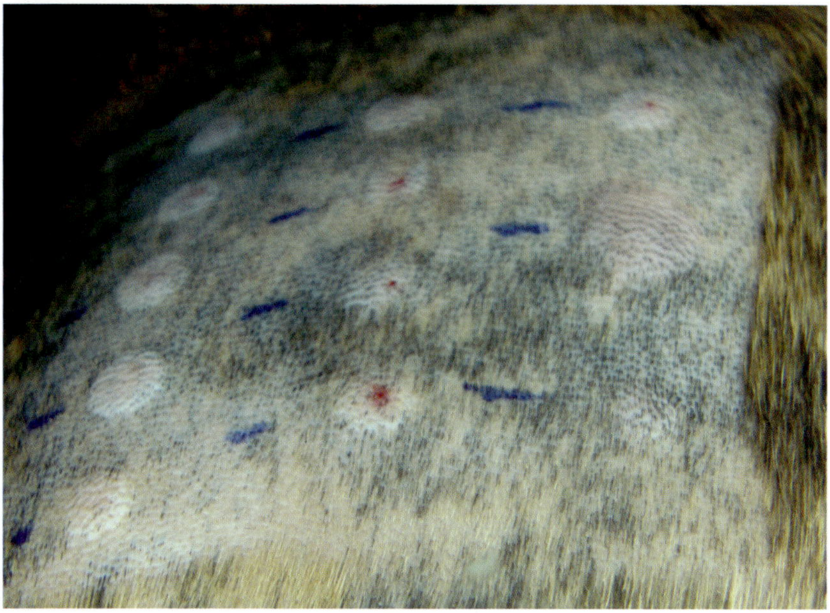

Figure 20. Intradermal skin reaction for allergy diagnosis in a dog.

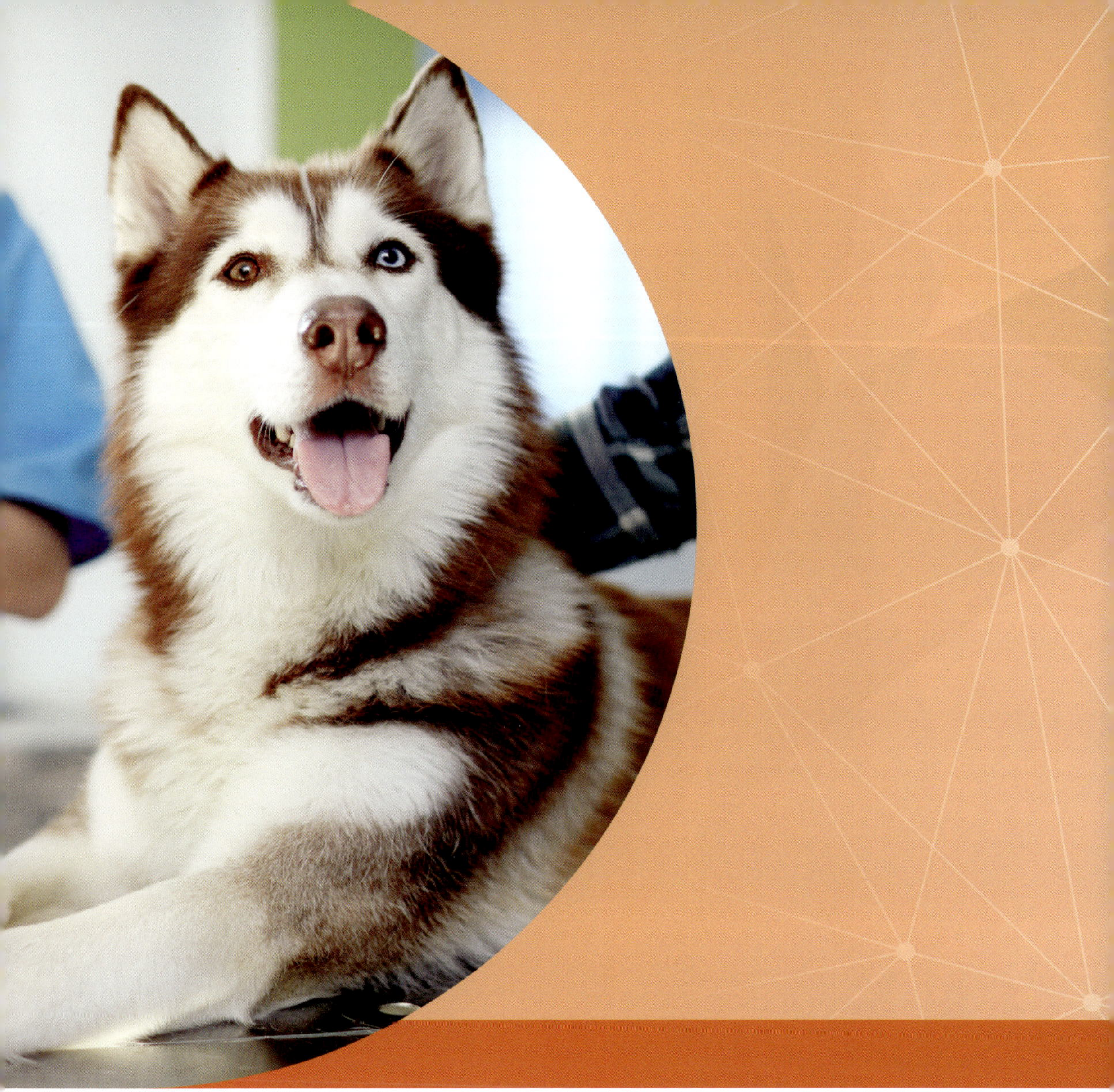

3

COMMUNICATION WITH CLIENTS

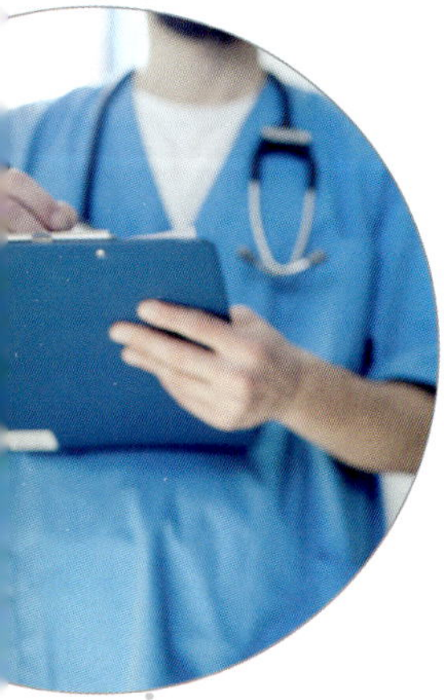

GOAL FOR CLIENTS:
100 % COMPREHENSION

In this internet age, with all the information that can be obtained using search engines and social networks, relationships with clients have changed enormously over the last decade.

The success or failure of a patient's treatment depends almost fully on the clinician–client relationship.

Veterinary surgeons must show empathy and convey a sense of security in the professional advice and experience-based knowledge they provide.

Owners must feel that their pet is unique in the treatment approach and value, as well as the diagnosis and the therapy offered.

Clients will trust a clinician who shows a personalised interest and provides information using understandable terminology.

It is very important for veterinary surgeons to understand how the general population converses about lesions and clinical signs. This can vary geographically, so it is important for them to master this terminology.

HOW TO EDUCATE CLIENTS

Spend as much time as necessary on obtaining the basic medical history. This should be done in a comfortable way in which the client feels that the veterinary surgeon is paying due attention.

In terms of business management, the profitability of these consultations is not a function of the time spent, but rather of the fees charged for it.

> The concept “there are no illnesses, just patients” is a premise to be understood by the owner from the outset.

The veterinary surgeon should emphasise the following aspects of allergies:

- These are usually chronic incurable diseases, but with a lot of dedication, they are fully controllable.
- It is not uncommon for the patient to occasionally suffer an acute episode, and the objective is to minimise these as much as possible.
- In regard to pruritus, we are not aiming to achieve a score of 0 (out of 10), but we aspire to achieve as low a score as possible to allow a good quality of life.

Treatment can be monitored based on the skin appearance and lesions, as well as on the comparison of pruritus scores. A score of 0 means the animal does not scratch at all, while a score of 10 means the animal does not sleep or eat because of scratching; a score of 5 means the animal responds to being called and stops scratching for a considerable period of time.

The owner, who lives with the patient on a daily basis, may propose a range of intermediate scores. Treatment can also be evaluated on a similar scale measuring the owner’s degree of satisfaction.

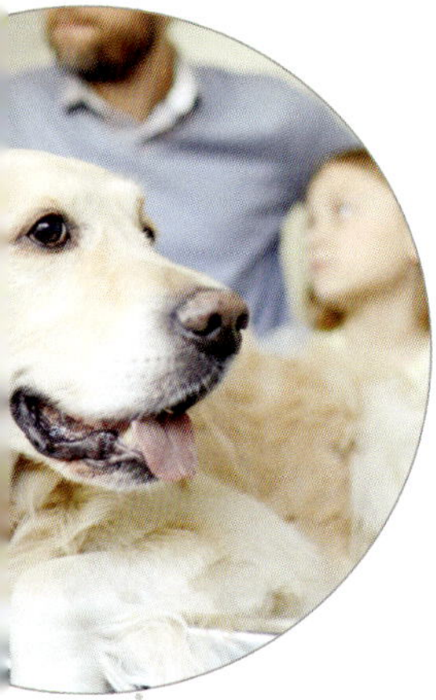

MANAGEMENT
OF DIFFERENT OWNER
ATTITUDES

Although the speciality is evolving, a range of client attitudes has been described and continues to exist.

Management of the ill patient must not change depending on the kind of owner, but veterinary surgeons must recognise that compliance depends on owners.

KINDS OF OWNERS

- The fully responsible and compliant owner.
- The owner who is tired or discouraged because of unsatisfactory results.
- The distrustful owner.
- The overwhelmed owner.
- The owner who comes out of obligation but does not have a major interest in their animal's problem.

CHARACTERISTICS
OF EACH KIND OF OWNER

FULLY RESPONSIBLE AND COMPLIANT

They usually bring an entire written history and follow instructions to the letter. They have a lot of faith in veterinary surgeons. Tip: Ask for the history on a pendrive and copy it, because it may be lengthy.

TIRED OR DISCOURAGED

They have already been to several clinics and the problem has not resolved. It is difficult to earn their trust, and the entire drug arsenal has already been administered to the patient. In these cases, it is essential to obtain as extensive a history as possible and, in some cases, start from zero.

DIFFICULT SITUATIONS
FOR THE OWNER RELATED TO
ALLERGY MANAGEMENT

It is very important for the vet to be aware of what they are asking or advising the patient's owner to do. They may not always be able to do everything proposed. For example:

- Comply strictly with an elimination diet.
- Bathe and dry a large, long-haired dog.
- Use a shampoo that does not lather.
- Administer pills to a cat.
- Measure how much water is drunk by a brachycephalic dog or by one of two dogs.
- Avoid feeding all stray cats that come to the door.
- Give "untouchable" cats anti-flea treatment.
- Tolerate polyuria from corticosteroids.
- Avoid feeding their animal "when it looks at them with those eyes".
- Understand terms such as interleukins, immunoglobulins, mast cells, pyoderma, etc.
- Understand that in general an excellent anti-flea product must be ingested by the flea for it to die.
- Understand that seawater is not good for the skin if salt is left without rinsing.
- Believe that shedding hair is normal and not necessarily pathological.

DISTRUSTFUL

They have read or will read everything on the internet. Their trust can be obtained with sincerity and knowledge. Everything must be in writing and recorded. It is possible to earn their trust quickly, but also to lose it.

OVERWHELMED

They are always watching the clock, and whilst explaining things to them, they keep checking their phone or use any excuse to leave the examination room. They may attend with children who distract them.

COMES OUT OF OBLIGATION

They are not concerned about their animal's problem, though the signs may bother them. They are expecting a miracle from us and as little work as possible. They will probably not comply with anything they have been instructed. It is essential to record everything instructed to the owner in the animal's medical record. These owners are usually pressured to visit the clinic by family or neighbours.

MOST COMMON ERRORS MADE BY THE VETERINARY SURGEON WHEN DEALING WITH THE OWNER
Speaking too technically.
Prejudging the client's financial resources.
Forgetting that many owners will check everything we have told them on the internet (or they have already done so).
Writing treatment plans without details.
Thinking that our opinion is unquestionable and forgetting that the groomer, breeder, pharmacist and neighbour will also voice an opinion.
Rushing through the consultation, taking too brief a history.
Administering an isoxazoline without taking a skin scrape first.
Administer treatments based on signs or lesions, without carefully considering possible diagnoses.
Forgetting to address the environment (fleas, *Sarcoptes*, dermatophytes, allergies).
Forgetting to consider the kind of owner (financial, cultural, social and family situation) when planning treatment.

DEEP-ROOTED MYTHS OWNERS MAY HARBOUR ABOUT ALLERGIES
Dogs cannot be bathed frequently.
Fleas are treated only in summertime.
Shampoo that does not lather is not good.
Immunotherapy is useless, based on prior experiences in the family.
A cat cannot have fleas if it never goes outside.
A cat does not scratch because it is never seen scratching. An animal licks a lot because it is grooming fastidiously.
An animal scratches a lot because of obsession or stress.
Administering a medicine for a long time, mainly an antibiotic, may be harmful to the animal.

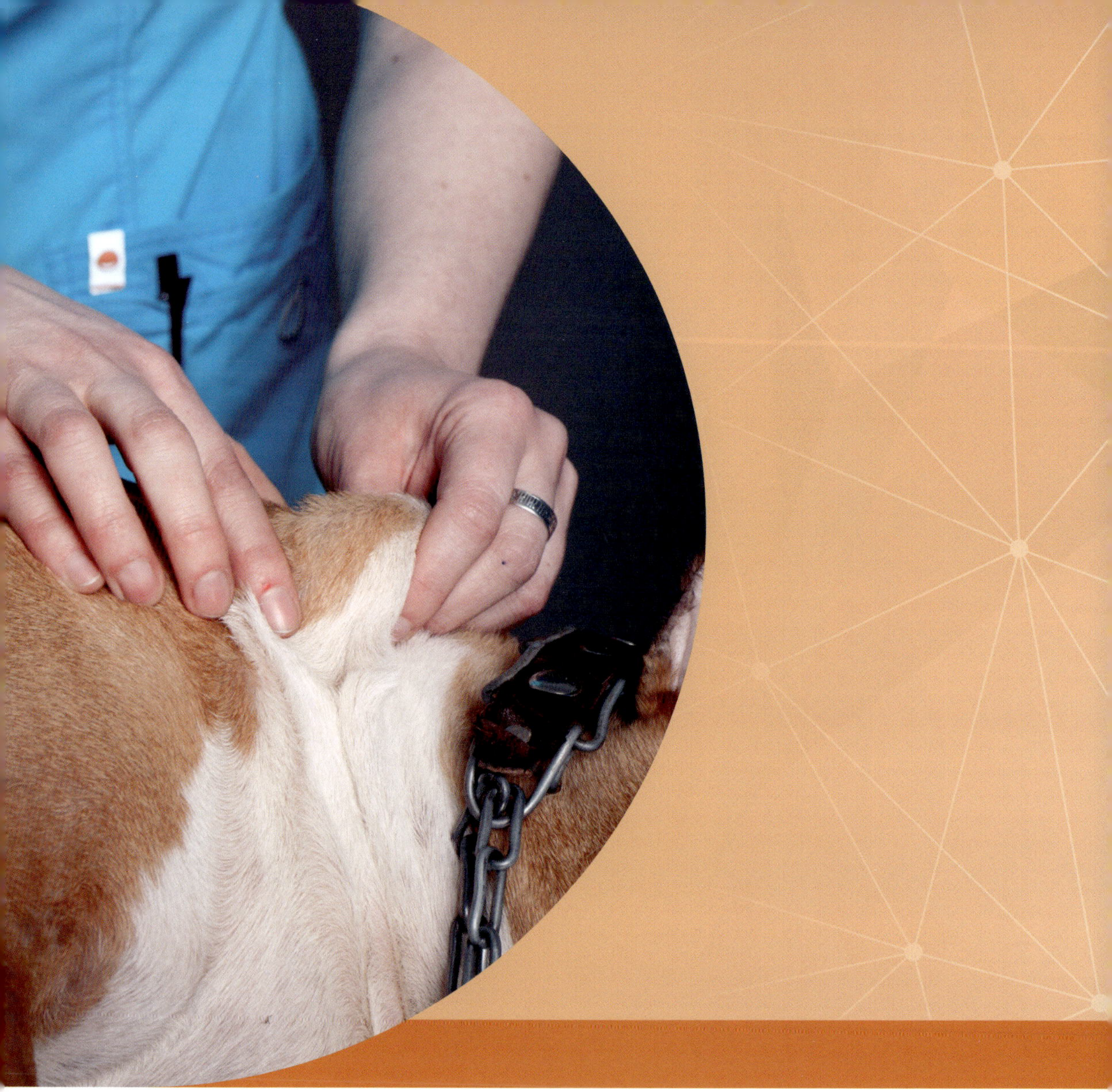

4

TREATMENT PROTOCOLS

The most common types of allergic dermatitis may be a combination of environmental, food and/or flea allergy and every aspect of the disease should be managed.

Other types of allergies may be easier to manage merely by avoiding the allergen, as in the case of contact dermatitis.

It is also worth remembering that each allergic individual expresses unique clinical signs, and the treatments and tools used vary by individual.

Just as these diseases are multifactorial, treatment entails several components.

The diagram below illustrates the four pillars of atopic dermatitis, mainly in dogs, according to recent studies (Fig. 1).

Different treatments are required according to the role of each of these factors in the disease; management is also different.

Figure 1. The four pillars of atopic dermatitis, mainly in dogs.

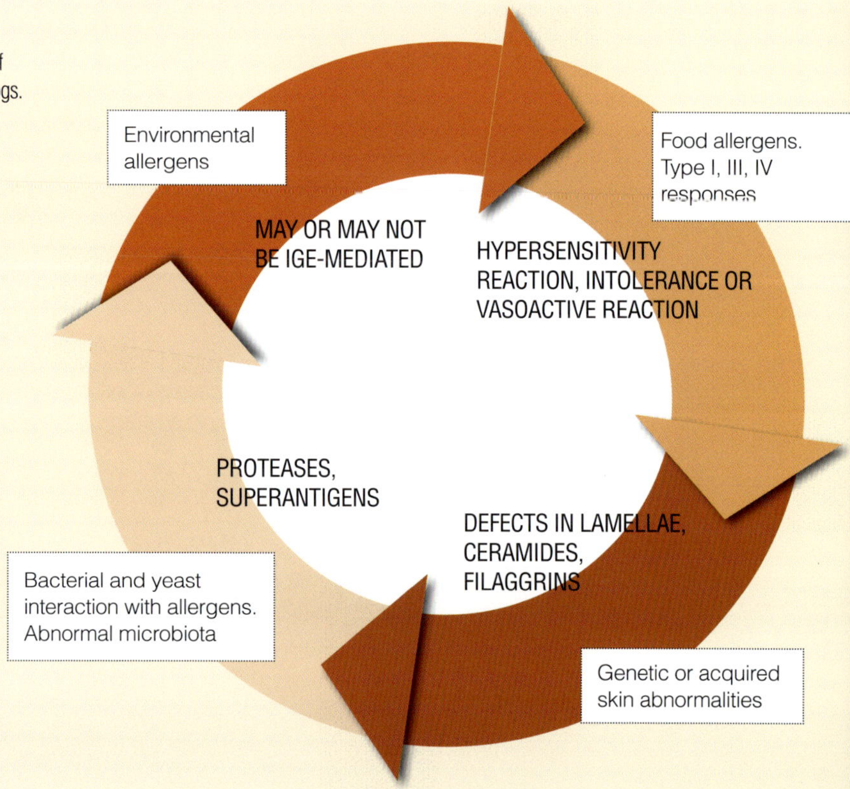

MANAGEMENT OF ACUTE
OR INITIAL EPISODES OF THE DISEASE

As with many other diseases, the severity of allergy signs varies. Specifically, some individuals with a very low allergy profile manifest only mild erythema and pruritus during certain times of the year; other individuals suffer from very severe signs that require intensive care (Fig. 2).

Allergic individuals are genetically predisposed to the disease, and the combination of certain "triggers" causes the initial signs to manifest or the relapse into an acute episode.

Allergic animals usually begin to show signs at an early age, although it is not uncommon to see individuals develop them at an older age. Animals that develop the first signs when older may be genetically predisposed but have not had sufficient exposure to trigger episodes. However, immunological abnormalities inherent to age, endocrine alterations, or sudden changes in the environment may cause the disease to manifest for the first time in these older patients.

Most commonly, the initial clinical signs of allergy occur between 6 months and 3 years of age*.

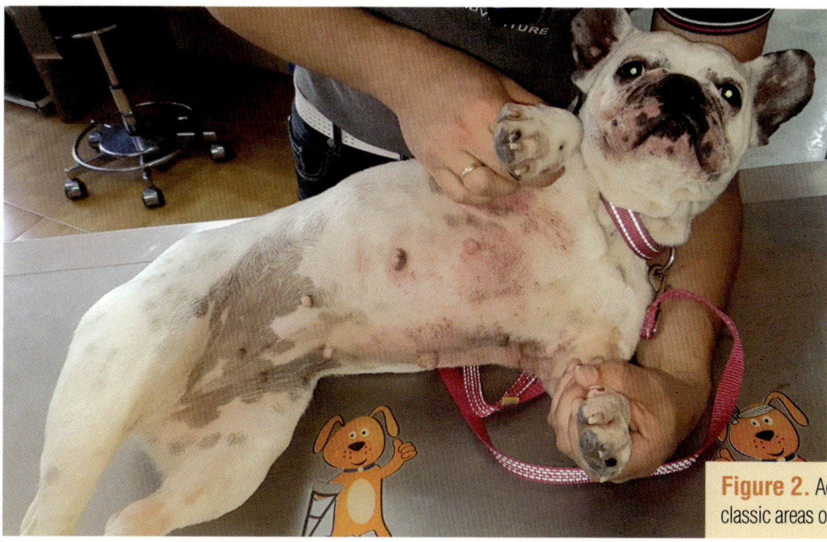

Figure 2. Acute episode. Note the classic areas of erythema.

*Although signs usually begin at one year of age, an increasing number of individuals are showing signs much earlier.

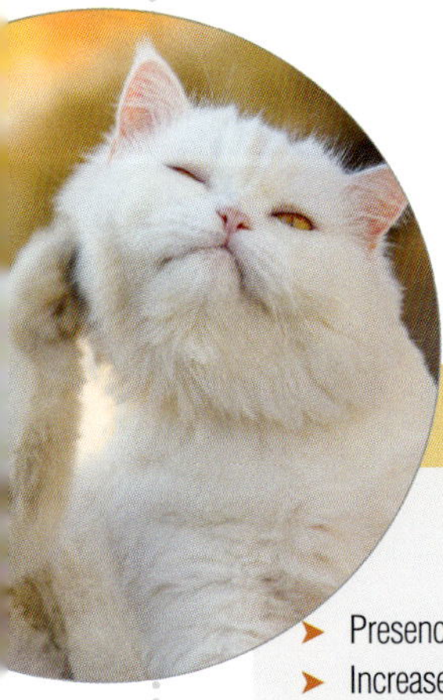

SEARCHING
FOR TRIGGERS

Triggers may induce an initial episode or a relapse in a controlled animal.

TRIGGERS OF ALLERGIC EPISODES

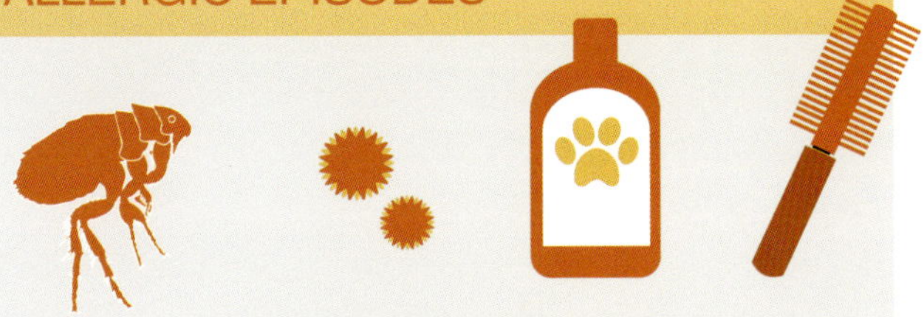

- Presence of fleas.
- Increased level of allergens:
  - Climate changes.
  - Habitat changes.
- Ingestion of a food allergen.
- Errors in managing a predisposed animal:
  - Poor rinsing of shampoo.
  - Drying with very hot air.
  - Not rinsing off salt after going into the sea.
  - Not rinsing off after going into a river with a lot of floating pollen.
  - Aggressive brushing.
  - Excessive or poor cleaning of the ears.
  - Removal of hair from the ears.
  - Not properly drying or cleaning the interdigital spaces in predisposed dogs after a walk.
- Sum or combination of several of these triggers.

It is often not possible to establish the precise cause or causes of a relapse, and in these cases, treatment can only be symptomatic. In situations in which the trigger is known, avoid it and take appropriate measures to treat the clinical signs.

For example, some patients retain skin moisture because of insufficient drying after bathing, which favours the development of pyotraumatic dermatitis. In these cases, the recommended treatment is topical substances such as antiseptic foam.

Many allergic animals can be controlled quite successfully with a diet that protects and replenishes the skin and the application of antiseptics and moisturisers that promote a natural and balanced microbiota.

As shown in the previous diagram (Fig. 1), the following is essential:

- Keep skin healthy, moisturised and structurally intact with topical treatments.
- Avoid allergens that may accumulate between the hair and skin.
- Control the microbiota so that microbial overgrowth does not occur.
- Offer a balanced diet that does not include known allergens, and/or provide nutraceuticals to maintain skin structure.
- Use the best anti-flea products available on the market without forgetting to treat the environment.

> Suitable shampoo therapy, correct anti-parasite application and a complete diet may help to achieve a successful treatment outcome.

USE OF ANTISEPTICS

The goal of antiseptics is to avoid the overgrowth of bacteria and yeasts, which is so common in these patients. Moreover, antiseptic use can obviate the need for antibiotics and thus prevent their indiscriminate use.

Antiseptics may be applied as sprays, shampoos or foams. Creams may also be used for very localised lesions. Some commercial spot-on formulations contain natural ingredients with a bacteriostatic and mycostatic function.

The skin must also be moisturised well, because xerosis is a significant problem that induces pruritus and microbial overgrowth in atopic animals. Towards this aim, shampoos are the ideal form of application.

MOST IMPORTANT SKIN ANTISEPTICS IN VETERINARY MEDICINE*
Chlorhexidine Very effective on fungi, viruses, and most bacteria.
Benzoyl peroxide Antibacterial effect. Degreasing effect and deep cleaning or flushing effect on the follicle.
Povidone-iodine Antibacterial and some antimycotic effect. Not very commonly used in veterinary products. There are some disadvantages such as staining and drying out.
Triclosan Disinfectant molecule with bactericidal and fungicidal effect.
Ethyl lactate Antibacterial with good penetration.
Phytosphingosine Restructuring and anti-inflammatory agent. This proceramide also acts as a natural antibacterial agent.
Piroctone olamine Anti-*Malassezia*, some antibacterial and keratoplastic effects.
Chloroxylenol (PCMX) Good antibacterial and fungicidal effect.
Hinokitiol Antibacterial.
Acetic acid 2 % – Boric acid 2 % Combined antibacterial and antifungal effect.
Selenium sulphide Keratomodulator, antiseptic action from release of sulphides.
Undecylenic acid Antimycotic, mainly.
Colloidal sulphur Bactericidal and fungicidal action from the release of sulphur and acidification. Acts as a keratomodulator.
Tris-EDTA Antibacterial effect and sensitiser to other antiseptics or antibiotics.
Peptides Synthetic peptides applied as a localised topical treatment or as a shampoo. May help to control bacteria and yeasts. The use of certain substances may also stimulate the production of natural peptides.
Hypochlorous acid Topically used antiseptic in the form of lotion or gel.

* The use of some azole derivatives and fusidic acid may boost the effects of the molecules mentioned.

SHAMPOO THERAPY

The goals of bathing allergic animals are as follows:

- Resolution of an infection.
- Avoiding the use of antibiotics.
- Treatment/prevention of recurrent infections.
- Antiseborrhoeic/keratomodulatory (keratoplastic/keratolytic).
- Antipruritic/anti-inflammatory.
- Moisturising/emollient.
- Odour removal.
- Allergen removal.
- Synergy with a systemic treatment.

Shampoo therapy aims to resolve acute episodes and to prevent relapses.

The use of ozone bubble baths may be recommended to facilitate absorption of products and as a soothing agent (Fig. 3).

Human shampoos with corticosteroids may be useful in some circumstances.

There are also skin restructuring substances that can be applied in the form of lotions or spot-on. These include ceramides, cholesterol, phytosphingosine, and fatty acids. Other products use extracts from different plant seeds with soothing and restructuring effects. Some of the most important are tea tree, rosemary, turmeric, oregano, and lavender.

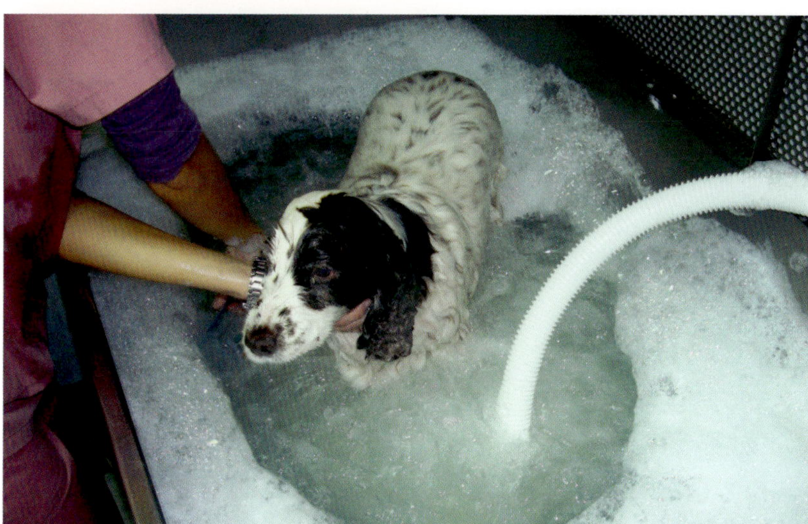

Figure 3. Ozone bubble baths to relieve pruritus.

Most common moisturising and soothing components of veterinary shampoos
Ceramides + omega fatty acids (restorative, hydrating, emollient)
Piroctone olamine (keratomodulator)
Phytosphingosine (anti-inflammatory, antiseborrhoeic)
Allantoin (hydrating agent)
Aloe/oat/salvia/*Epilobium* (anti-inflammatory, hydrating)
Sodium lauryl ether sulphate, menthol, peppermint, zinc gluconate (soothing agents)
Glycerine, propylene glycol, urea derivatives (hydrating agents)

Most common components to treat keratinisation disorders
Salicyclic acid (dry seborrhoea)
Sulphur
Selenium sulphide
Benzoyl peroxide
Ammonium lactate
Ethyl lactate
Zinc gluconate (oily seborrhoea)
Vitamin B_6
Phytosphingosine
Essential fatty acids
Glycerine–propylene glycol
Lactic acid
Polyester fatty acids
Epilobium (keratomodulator)

Most common antiseptic components in veterinary shampoos
Chlorhexidine
Benzoyl peroxide
Povidone-iodine
Hinokitiol
Triclosan
Chloroxylenol
Ethyl lactate
Phytosphingosine
Piroctone olamine
Miconazole
Ketoconazole
Epilobium
Colloidal sulphur
Peptides
Plant-derived defensins

Most common anti-pruritogenic components in veterinary shampoos
Colloidal oat flour
Wheat germ oil
Aloe derivatives
Menthol
Sage extract
Epilobium angustifolium
Lipid complexes and ceramide derivatives

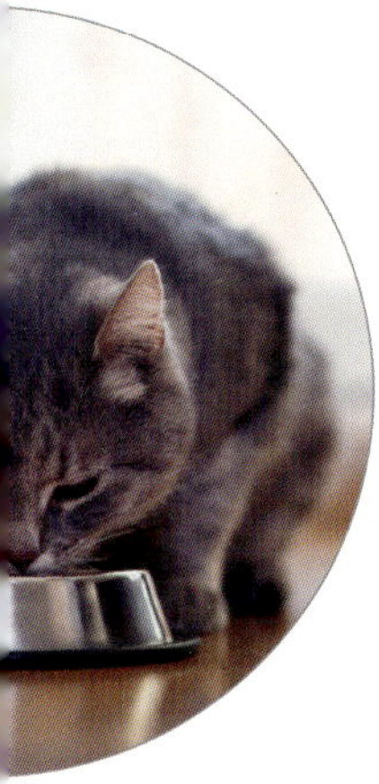

DIET

A correct diet is essential in animals with allergy and skin deficiencies such as a defective skin structure – defective lipid lamellae; filaggrin or ceramide deficiency –, with consequent dehydration of the skin. A proper diet is also very important for food allergies; if a food allergen is identified, it should be removed from the diet to provide relief.

A suitable level of omega-3 and -6 fatty acids, nutraceuticals that improve skin quality and soothe pruritus, quality packaging that keeps the food insect-free, and high quality proteins are key to improving skin health.

In some cases, the owner should be encouraged to buy small packages to avoid the degradation of the product over time. Along the same lines, it may be very useful to store the food in small portions within sealed plastic containers that can be frozen to avoid an infestation.

If the allergenic proteins are known, foods free of these proteins must be selected.

One way to guarantee a proper diet is by using hydrolysed proteins.

Many of the substances found in high quality food may also be provided by nutritional supplements. There are currently some excellent products of this kind that provide all the components necessary to restore the skin's structural integrity and immune function. These include essential fatty acids, nucleotides, hyaluronic acid, zinc, and antioxidants such as vitamin E.

STEPS TO DETERMINE
WHETHER A PROTEIN INDUCES
AN ADVERSE REACTION

STEP 1

Undertake an "elimination diet" using hydrolysed or novel proteins.

After 8 to 10 weeks of this diet and confirming that there has been no relapse in the patient without another preventive treatment, move on to step 2.

STEP 2

Undertake the "challenge diet". This is usually the only way of confirming the allergenic potential of proteins.

Approximately every 10 days, the individual is challenged with a new protein for just one day, keeping the food from the elimination diet as the base diet.

Proteins usually tested are from chicken, beef, dairy products, eggs, pork, white fish, blue fish and soya.

After 10 days without any obvious relapse, move on to the next protein.

If any protein causes a relapse, it can be controlled or slowed with oclacitinib. Once the patient has recovered from the pruritus and lesions, the test can be continued.

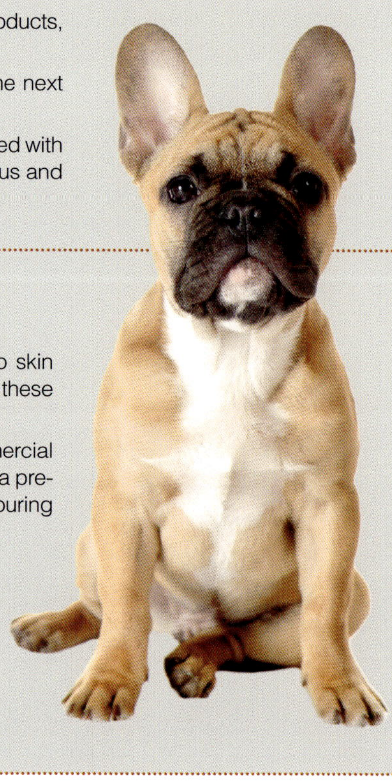

STEP 3

If, after testing all the proteins named above, there is no skin reaction, the animal is determined not to have AFRs to these common proteins.

If any kind of relapse occurs when reintroducing a commercial food product and it is confirmed that environmental and flea prevention conditions have not varied, a preservative or colouring agent in the food product may be suspected.

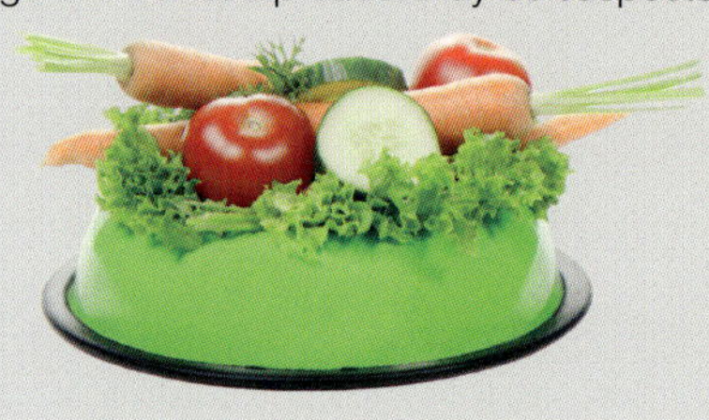

CONTROL OF PRURITUS

It is essential to break the vicious cycle of pruritus–inflammation–infection.

In addition to the treatments mentioned above, others are currently available to manage pruritus and control inflammation and infection, either directly or indirectly.

When an infection becomes deep, there is no solution other than to use antibiotics and, in the case of *Malassezia*, antifungal agents. For superficial infections, the empirical recommendation is first-generation beta-lactam antibiotics such as cephalexin or cefadroxil, or amoxicillin with clavulanic acid.

The use of antiseptics is sufficient in most cases to control *Malassezia* and bacteria and to reduce inflammation. However, in other cases, azoles such as ketoconazole, itraconazole, and fluconazole must be used in dogs; itraconazole should be used in cats. Terbinafine may also be a good treatment option.

Oclacitinib, at a short-term initial dose, and subsequently at a maintenance dose, is an excellent control measure for pruritus and an anti-inflammatory. When inflammation is extensive, as in the case of stenotic ear canals or very inflamed interdigital spaces, the use of prednisone, prednisolone or methylprednisolone is also indicated.

Once an allergic episode or the initial signs of the disease are controlled, discontinue the oclacitinib to observe the individual's response without superinfections and inflammation.

Shampoo therapy combined with a correct diet and preventive environmental measures may often be sufficient, but in some cases antipruritogenic agents must be used repeatedly.

At this time we must consider the use of maintenance or follow-up medication (oclacitinib, cyclosporine, lokivetmab).

In cats, episodes may involve a reaction pattern or a combination of patterns. Options from the "therapeutic arsenal" are a diet that favours healthy skin, good flea prevention, and short-term corticosteroids. A wider variety of corticosteroids may be used for acute episodes in cats because efficacy varies by individual. For example, some individuals improve with prednisolone or dexamethasone and others with prednisone. Some fractious cats may require injectable methylprednisolone acetate.

Regarding antibiotics for cats, the guidelines are the same as in dogs, but cefovecin is often used for fractious cats.

MAINTENANCE
OF THE CONTROLLED PATIENT

Patients with controlled pruritus, a good quality of life, and healthy-looking skin require maintenance measures including nutrition and, in some cases, medication for lengthy periods or for life.

Maintenance is based on the use of an appropriate shampoo with the necessary frequency to hydrate the skin and balance the microbiota, as well as on diet or supplements that support skin metabolism. The most common long-term maintenance medications in dogs, depending on the severity of the case and treatment response, are as follows:

- Oclacitinib.
- Cyclosporine.
- Lokivetmab.

Palmitoylethanolamide (PEA) may be a useful nutraceutical in controlled dogs to hinder the migration of mast cells and help avoid recurrence of the disease.

In very severe cases, combinations of different medicines and sometimes individualised doses may be necessary.

Each patient is completely different, and our skill as veterinary clinicians is combining the type of patient and owner with the clinical signs to find the drug with the most suitable characteristics for the case. For example, some canine patients are perfectly managed for short or longer periods with oclacitinib tablets. Other owners prefer the convenience of a monthly injection of lokivetmab to control topical pruritus. In other cases, the use of cyclosporine is preferred, and it is used every two days for immunomodulation.

Some patients tend to develop initial signs in particular regions of the body such as the interdigital spaces or the ears. There are topical veterinary preparations with corticosteroids in the form of sprays and creams that can slow down the development of these signs. The use of antiseptic wipes may stop microbial overgrowth in these areas.

Proactive treatment with topical corticosteroids may slow the development of otitis or pododermatitis.

They can be used preventively twice a week, for example. Corticosteroids can be very useful but should be used in moderation, preferably topically. If they must be used systemically to control an episode, there is a very useful formula to calculate the maximum annual dose of prednisone or prednisolone for a dog: the animal's weight multiplied by 30 gives the total dose in milligrams that can be administered each year. For example, for a dog weighing 10 kg: $10 \times 30 = 300$ mg. This is the maximum amount of corticosteroids that can be administered in one year.

The basis for control of an allergic cat is also diet, supplements and topical products. Logically, fleas must be avoided.

Cyclosporine is widely used, either alone or combined with different products such as antihistamines and palmitoylethanolamide.

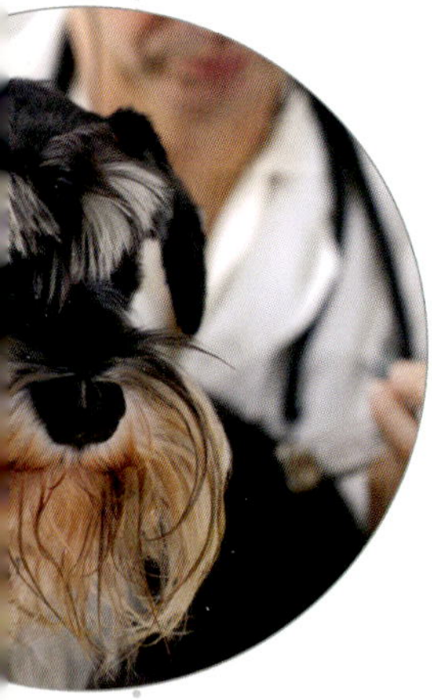

IMMUNOTHERAPY

The determination of environmental allergens involved in atopic dermatitis may be useful to avoid them or to design desensitising immunotherapy.

The success of desensitisation depends on the correct identification of the allergens to subsequently administer immunotherapy, whether subcutaneously or orally.

As a general recommendation, immunotherapy should be administered for at least for one year before deciding whether it is effective and should be continued.

Not all dogs improve significantly, but many dogs do have fewer episodes over the year.

This may also be a useful approach for cats, but diagnostic methods are somewhat more variable.

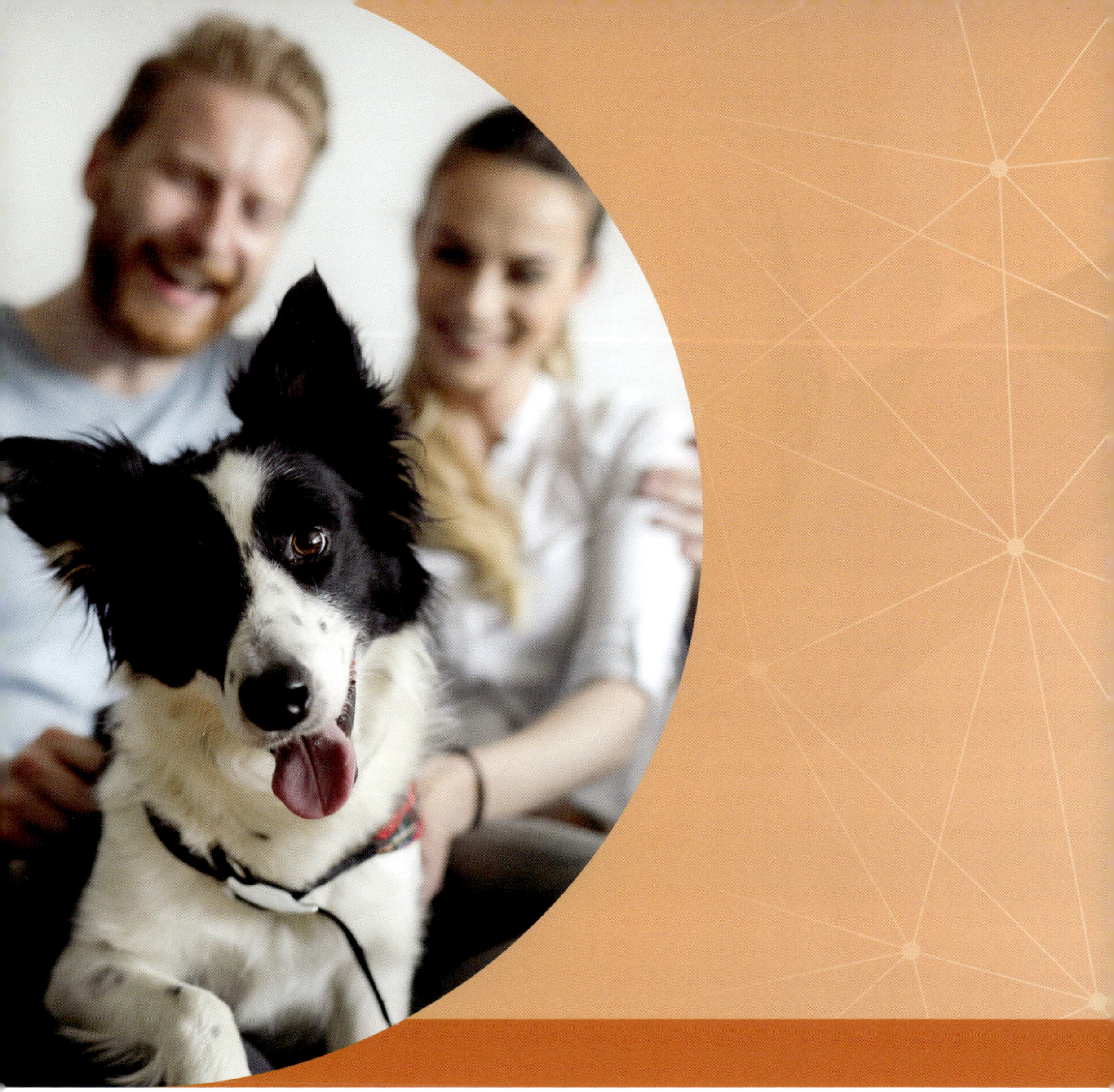

5

RECOMMENDATIONS FOR THE OWNER: FOLLOW-UP

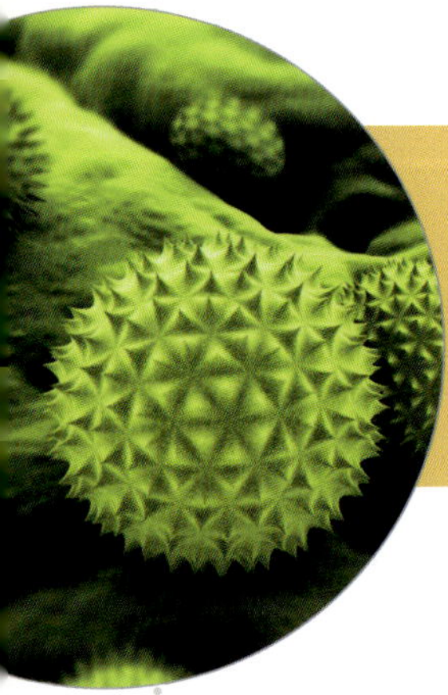

TIP

Tell the owner that allergies may not be curable because they are exaggerated reactions with a genetic basis. The patient can be controlled only if the allergen is avoided, if they are desensitised, or if clinical signs are treated with various drugs.

THE IMPORTANCE
OF DIET

A balanced and top-quality diet is important for all patients, regardless of whether they suffer from skin problems. However, a correct diet is critically important in those animals with dermatitis and allergies. If we recall that these patients, mainly dogs, can have cutaneous structural deficiencies that lead to xerosis and superinfections, foods that improve skin structure will be essential as a support for treatment.

Different components are available and include plant extracts, essential omega 3 and 6 fatty acids, special proteins, nucleotides, antioxidants, phytonutrients, vitamins, and other substances that help to restructure the skin of atopic individuals and may be provided by food products or supplements.

The owner must be informed that this kind of commercial diet not only "feeds" their pet but also "treats" the disease.

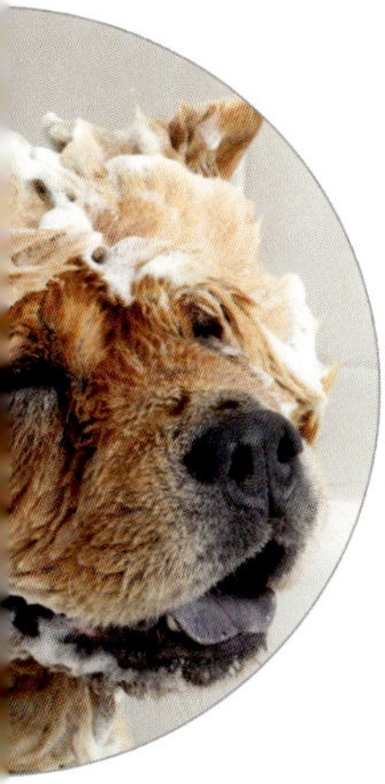

SHAMPOO THERAPY
AND HYDRATION THERAPY

Owners must understand that shampoo has not only cleansing and beautifying functions, but also a skin treatment function.

Shampoo functions can be summarised as follows:

- Part of an overall treatment.
- Single treatment.
- Aesthetic or simple cleansing purposes.
- Hydration/moisturising.
- Keratomodulation.
- Elimination of allergens.
- Relief for pruritus and inflammation.
- Antisepsis.

Shampoo baths use water to disseminate and facilitate penetration of various ingredients with certain known functions.

Thanks to surfactant agents and other components, shampoos can bind lipophilic and hydrophilic substances with different electrostatic charges, thus enabling water to wash them out. In some cases, the substances contained in shampoos may help the skin retain water and thus offer a moisturising and emollient effect.

Shampoo therapy involves certain terms that must be explained correctly to the owner:

Moisturiser	Retains surface water
Hydrating agent	Prevents evaporation of deep water
Emollient	Softens hard areas and increases flexibility
Keratolytic agent	Degrades or removes keratin
Keratoplastic agent	Activates cornification of keratinocytes
Restructuring agent	Repair, seals and softens

Veterinary clinicians should be familiar with the different shampoo ingredients involved:

- Surface active agents, or surfactants (cleansers, foaming agents and conditioners).
- Thickeners (facilitate application of the product).
- Softeners.
- Preservatives.
- Perfumes.
- Pearlising agents (wax).
- Occasional additives, colouring agents and opacifiers.
- Component vehicles: liposomes, microspheres.
- Therapeutic components if included.

It is very important to understand the mechanism of each shampoo and instruct owners that a lather may need to act on the body for 10 minutes to perform all these actions.

Shampoo therapy can also be very important in cats. Its use should be considered for an owner with a cooperative patient.

Certain components may be irritants and not indicated in cats, but some may be used with certain restrictions.

> For allergic cats, it is also important to keep the hair short year-round.

GUIDELINES FOR MANAGEMENT

- Two applications of the shampoo; the second application should be left for approximately 10 minutes to enhance action of the active substances.
- Next, soak and rinse for at least 5 minutes to avoid irritation and allow the skin to suitably hydrate. Do not overlook the ventral part of the body.
- Frequency: several times per week (generally two) for at least 2 weeks. The frequency may be decreased later, depending on the specific case, normally to 1–2 week intervals.
- The mechanical effect of bathing (removal of scales and scabs) is always beneficial.
- Water hydrates the stratum corneum, but this effect is temporary in the absence of hydrating agents.
- Shampoo may be used in a limited area or over the entire body.
- Drying with hot air can reactivate pruritus, which can induce xerosis. Therefore, use gentle, lukewarm air or a towel. Portable cold-air dryers must be used at a suitable distance to avoid drying out the skin.

THE IMPORTANCE OF
AVOIDING SKIN PARASITES

While parasites can affect any animal through their presence and life cycle, the skin of allergic animals is much more sensitive to them, so they should be avoided as much as possible.

Concerning allergic diseases, fleas are the parasite ***par excellence*** because in both cats and dogs, they multiply the effects of allergies and push the animal to the pruritus threshold. Studies confirm that atopic animals are usually more allergic to flea bites than nonatopic animals; thus, in atopic patients, we must choose the best methods currently available.

Every adult flea represents a large number of juvenile fleas in the animal's environment, so treatment should be global.

- The best way to keep skin hydrated is by applying moisturising sprays before drying the whole animal, which enables the skin to retain water from the rinse.
- It is recommended to keep hair less than 5 cm long. This will ease bathing and will avoid accumulation of allergens.

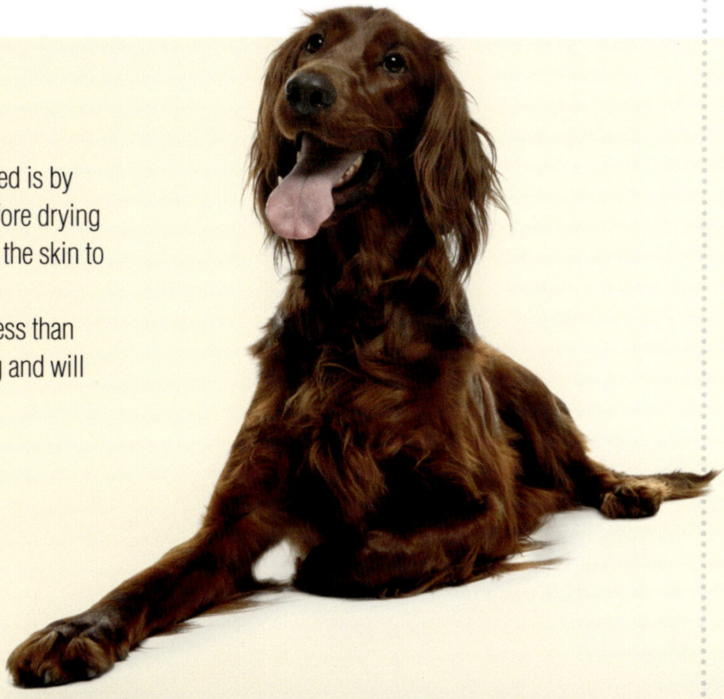

Different sprays and foggers containing juvenile development inhibitors are available to treat the environment. Some substances applied to the animal act on the complete flea life cycle (e.g. on eggs and larvae).

Adulticides are contained in sprays, collars, spot-ons, and oral tablets. Efficacy depends on their quality and level of infestation of the environment. There are circumstances in which combinations of two or more products may be necessary for actual eradication of the parasite (Fig. 1).

Nevertheless, preventing all flea bites in allergic animals remains a challenge.

Most commonly used products
Pyrethrins
Fipronil and its derivatives
Imidocarb
Indoxacarb
Dinotefuran
Nitenpyram
Spinosad
Isoxazolines
Spinetoram

When considering differential diagnoses we must never overlook the possibility of *Sarcoptes*, *Cheyletiella* and, often, ticks. The first two parasites induce significant pruritus, and ticks may induce pyotraumatic dermatitis, even though they are not a primary cause.

In cats, *Notoedres*, *Cheyletiella* and, to a lesser extent, ticks, must also be considered. In the last few years there has been a major evolution in spot-ons for cats containing isoxazolines and/or macrocyclic lactones, which make them very effective against ticks and other insects.

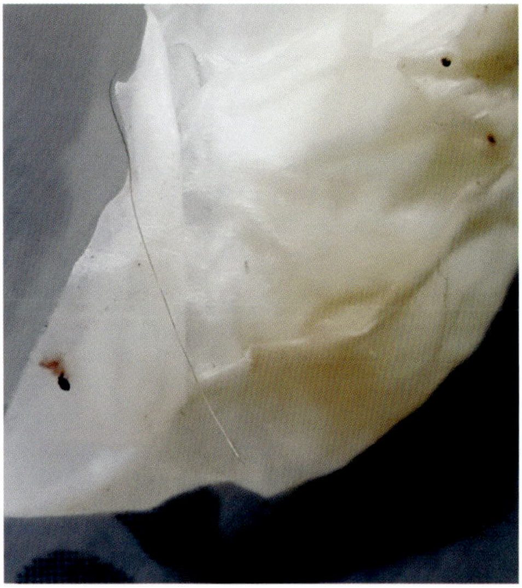

Figure 1. Presence of flea faeces, confirmed by brushing onto moist paper. Very common trigger of an episode.

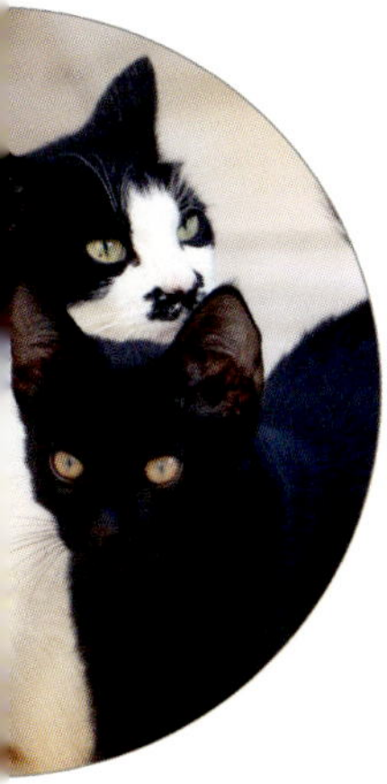

GENERAL PREVENTIVE MEASURES

As this guide has emphasised, communication with the owner is essential for conveying information and achieving compliance with treatments and management of the allergic animal.

Without the cooperation of owners it is impossible to manage the treatment of allergic patients.

Certain general recommendations must be conveyed to the owner, regardless of the allergen. This advice is essential from the very first visit.

PREVENTIVE MEASURES FOR DOG AND CAT OWNERS
Try not to clean the house in the animal's presence.
Avoid vacuuming and changing the vacuum bag or air conditioning filters near the patient.
Always use ceramic or metal food and water dishes (avoid plastic).
Use bagless vacuums or steam cleaners.
Wear designated clothes around allergic patients and launder them frequently.
Try to ensure that dry food is kept in dry areas and vacuum-sealed if possible. Small bags that are consumed quickly are recommended. In the case of cats, consider giving wet food in accordance with the allergy tests.
Dehumidifiers may be recommended as needed.
Be watchful for the start of any episode (Fig. 2). The previous chapter describes the triggers that the owner must be familiar with to avoid the animal injuring itself and developing reaction patterns.
Avoid contact with stray cats. Avoid feeding stray cats in the patient's environment (they may have fleas).

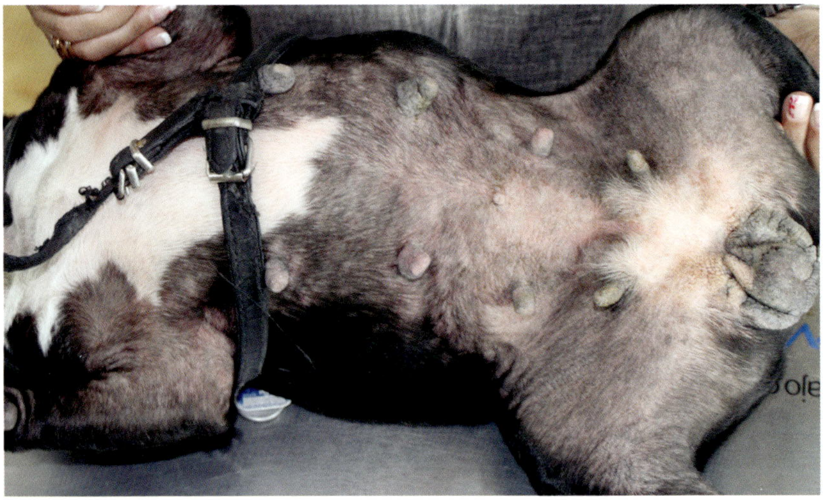

Figure 2. Note the erythema signalling an acute episode in a relatively well-controlled animal with chronic skin abnormalities.

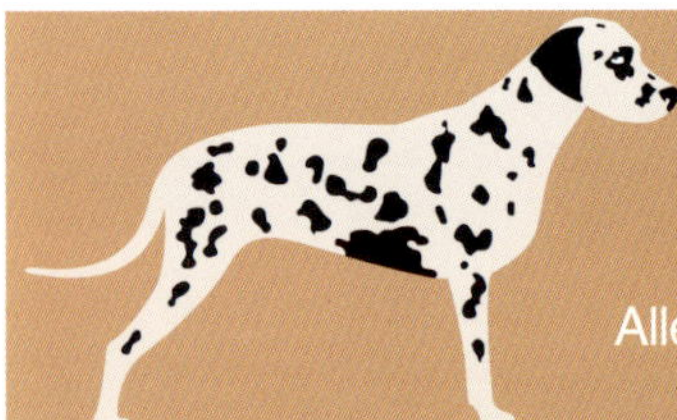 Allergic dog	Allergic cat 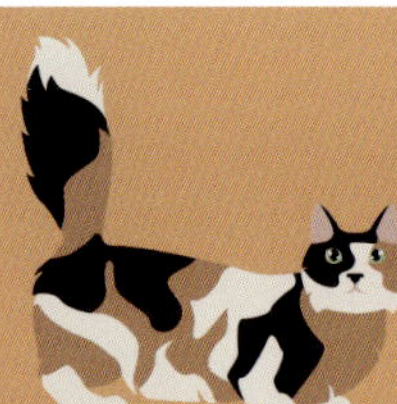
Try to avoid allowing the animal on recently mown grass.	Enrich the environment with scratching posts, hiding places and toys. Consider use of environmental pheromones.
Rinse the animal after it goes in a sea or river to avoid retaining dissolved pollen or salt.	Note changes in behaviour and remember that scratching is much less obvious in cats.
After a walk, remove pollen from the skin with a wet cloth.	Fleas can enter the house even if the cat never goes outside.
Keep hair short year-round, if possible, less than 5 cm long.	Keep hair short year-round.
Wipe sensitive areas with antiseptic wipes even just once a day (between the digits, axillae, groin and ears).	
Avoid walks on windy days at times when pollen counts are high. These are usually 7 to 10 a.m. and 7 to 10 p.m., depending on the plants in the area and the season.	

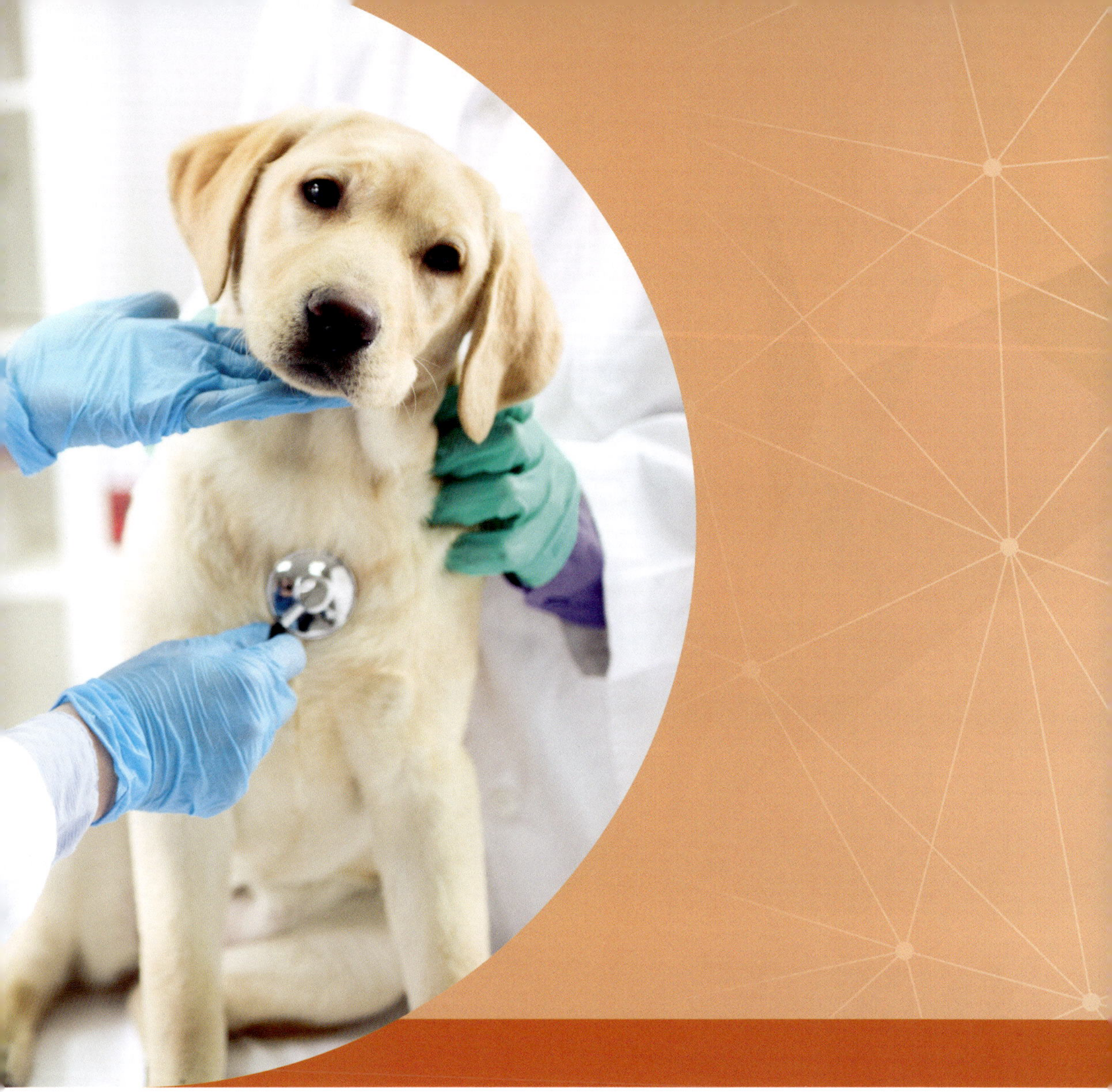

6

CASE STUDIES: EXPERIENCE-BASED MEDICINE

CASE STUDY 1

FELINE HYPERSENSITIVITY

This case features much of what is mentioned in this guide. The progression may vary depending on factors such as the specific characteristics of the animal and owner.

PATIENT SIGNALMENT

SPECIES:	CAT
BREED:	DOMESTIC SHORTHAIR
SEX:	MALE
AGE:	2 YEARS
WEIGHT:	3 KG

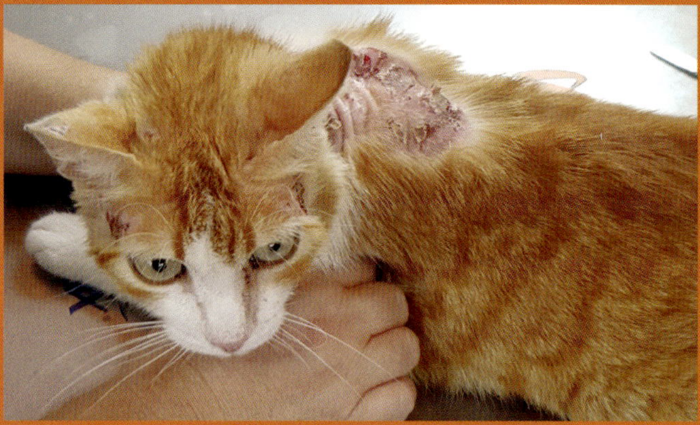

HISTORY

The patient lives in a flat with access to a terrace where it may have contact with a neighbouring cat. Vaccination and endoparasite prevention have been performed correctly. Flea prevention has been performed irregularly, but no fleas have ever been seen.

The patient is taken to the clinic with acute allergic signs. The animal has suffered similar signs previously but never as severely as on this occasion.

IMPORTANT QUESTIONS
TO ASK THE OWNER WHEN OBTAINING A HISTORY

1. Has anyone in the family had problems with insect bites?
2. Describe how your animal scratches.
3. Describe the environment in which the animal lives.
4. Does the animal have direct or indirect contact with other animals?
5. When was the last time you saw fleas on your animal?
6. What is the animal's diet and what do its stools look like?
7. Has the animal ever been treated for these problems, and which medication was administered?

ANALYSIS OF THE QUESTIONS

1. Has anyone in the family had problems with insect bites?

It is important to look for other ways to detect fleas. In feline medicine, owners often do not see fleas because of the intensity and agility with which cats groom themselves and remove them. Some owners associate the presence of fleas with the lack of housecleaning, so be very careful when asking about this topic.

2. Describe how your animal scratches

The way in which a patient scratches may suggest the origin of the pruritus. In cats there is a clear predominance of licking, which may vary in intensity and become compulsive. Sometimes cats chew and pull out their hair, and less often they scratch with their legs like dogs. A cat's compulsive search for areas to chew may indicate flea bites.

3. Describe the environment in which your animal lives

In feline medicine, it is very important to focus on the environment and the cat's interaction with it, because a deficient environment may give rise to behavioural abnormalities.

Verify the presence of sufficient scratching posts and suitable ground-level and elevated hiding places. Ensure there are enough litter boxes. One more litter box than the number of cats is appropriate. These questions will help to analyse the cat's psychological health and differentiate compulsive behaviour from true pruritus.

4. Does your animal have direct or indirect contact with other animals?

Fleas can enter the home by different routes even if the cat never goes outside. People coming in may have fleas on their clothing, and visiting animals may also bring the parasite into the cat's environment. In this case, access to a terrace may allow temporary contact with other cats from neighbouring areas.

5. When was the last time you saw fleas on your animal?

All these questions highlight the importance of ruling out fleas. This is because flea allergy dermatitis is the first differential diagnosis in areas where fleas are present. Moreover, these insects can go undetected by owners. Although owners may state they have seen no fleas, this question does not directly address the actual presence of fleas but allows the owner freedom to "confess" that they have seen some. If fleas were present in the past, juvenile forms may remain.

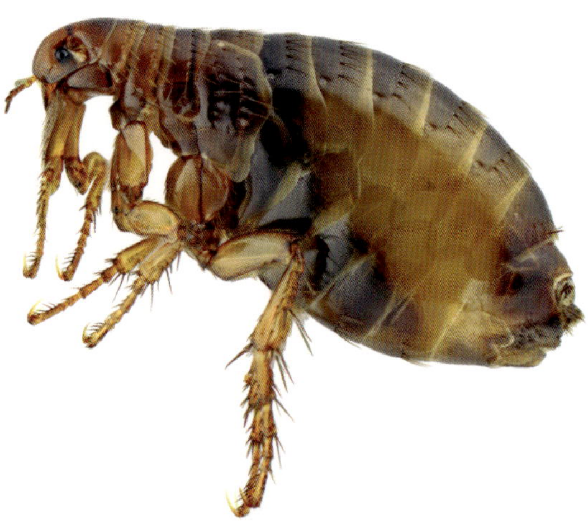

6. What is your animal's diet and what does its stool look like?

   This question is related to gastrointestinal health and its common relationship with skin problems. In dogs, this question is essential; in cats, this is less relevant because gastrointestinal problems related to food allergies with skin signs are not as common. Knowing about their diet will assist in designing a future elimination diet. The ingredients eaten and food type (dry or wet) are important.

7. Has the animal ever been treated for these problems, and which medication was administered?

   This question is very important as it reveals the response to previous treatments and suggests certain diagnoses.

SUMMARY OF ANSWERS

- The owner confirms that they have not seen fleas, that they use spot-ons occasionally, and that the animal mainly eats dry food, although the animal also accepts wet food if offered.
- The owner believes there is no contact with neighbouring animals although they have heard some meowing on a few nights.
- The environment is appropriate in that the feeding and drinking area is separated from the litter boxes. There are different hiding places and sufficient scratching posts.
- The owner tells us that the problem is palpable "little spots", and that once a veterinary surgeon gave the animal an injection that made them go away.
- When scratching, the animal uses its hindlimb to reach the area and then licks a lot afterwards.

DIAGNOSTIC APPROACH

General examination: no obvious abnormalities.

Dermatological examination: localised alopecia in the cervical and interscapular area together with supraocular lesions. Different-sized scabs, erythema, and signs of excoriation can be observed (Fig. 1). Some pain when touched.

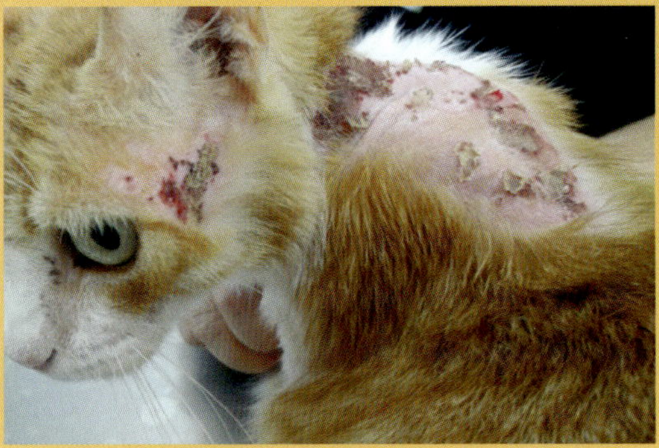

Figure 1. Patient's condition at presentation.

DIFFERENTIAL DIAGNOSES

These lesions correspond to two of the reaction patterns in cats: head and neck dermatitis and miliary dermatitis.

These patterns may appear in many pathologies, summarised as follows:

1. Head and neck dermatitis

- Pulicosis–FAD.
- Mosquito bites.
- Food allergy.
- Atopic-like hypersensitivity.
- Bacteria and *Malassezia*.
- Demodicosis.
- Notoedric mange.
- Otoacariasis.
- Trombiculiasis.
- Dermatophytosis.
- Dirty face syndrome.
- Others.

2. Miliary dermatitis

- Presence of fleas or flea allergy (more than 75 % of cases).
- Hypersensitivity to food products.
- Atopic-like hypersensitivity.
- Hypersensitivity to mosquito bites.
- Notoedric mange.
- Demodicosis.
- *Otodectes*.
- Psychogenic dermatitis.
- Pediculosis.
- Trombiculiasis.
- Dermatophytosis.
- Others.

The differential diagnoses clearly overlap.

If six Favrot's criteria are met, we can conclude with high specificity that this is an atopic patient (see page 53).

By combining this analysis with additional tests and therapeutic diagnostics, we can reach a definitive diagnosis.

The most important additional tests are skin scrapes, cytology of scabs, Wood's lamp examination, and trichogram. The aim is to look for parasites, dermatophytes, and broken hairs that confirm a self-induced aetiology. Looking under scabs reveals the kind of inflammation and identifies possible infectious agents.

The skin scrape results were negative. The trichogram revealed hairs with a broken tip. The Wood's lamp did not fluoresce the lesions.

Response to corticosteroids may help to rule out psychogenic alopecia. In this case, the lesion is highly inflammatory, ruling out a solely behavioural origin.

FAVROT'S CRITERIA

		YES	NO
1.	Presence of pruritus since the onset of the problem	✓	
2.	Presence of at least two of the following clinical signs: › Symmetrical alopecia › Crusted papular dermatitis or miliary dermatitis › Plaque and nodular dermatitis (lesions of the feline eosinophilic granuloma complex) › Erosions or ulcers in the cervical or facial region	✓	
3.	At least two locations affected	✓	
4.	Miliary dermatitis as the predominant pattern	✓	
5.	Eosinophilic dermatitis, symmetrical alopecia, or erosions or ulcers in the region of the neck, head, lips, or ears	✓	
6.	Nonsymmetrical alopecia in the dorsocaudal region, tail, or hindlimbs		✗
7.	Symmetrical alopecia on the abdomen		✗
8.	No erosions or ulcers on the forelimbs	✓	
9.	No lesions in the axillary or sternal regions	✓	
10.	No nodules or tumours	✓	

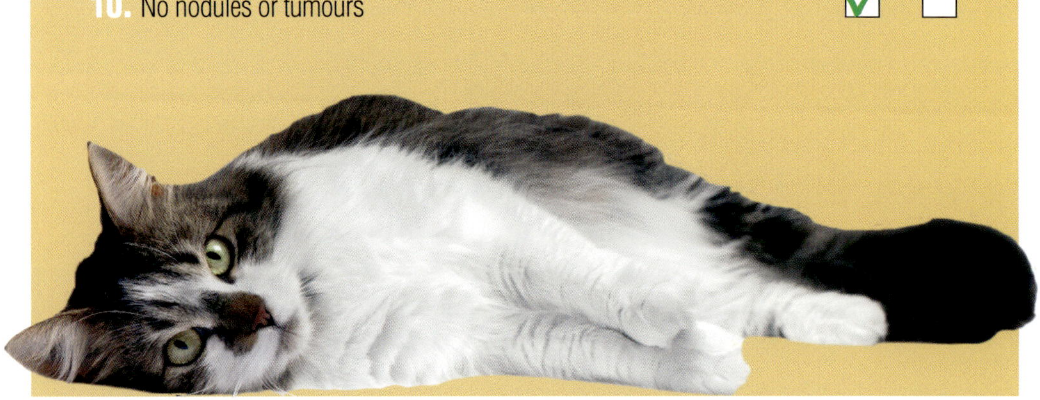

DISCUSSION

Cytology confirms the presence of granulocytes, mainly eosinophils (Fig. 2).

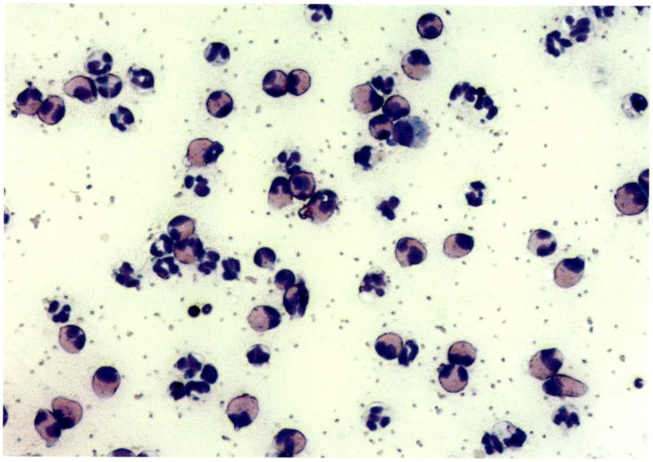

Figure 2. Eosinophilic inflammatory cytology seen under scab.

This suggests primarily eosinophilic miliary dermatitis, which, together with the other negative test results and the eight positive Favrot's criteria, leads to considering an allergy.

To rule out the role of fleas, we must give highly effective anti-flea agents and treat the environment.

Once fleas are controlled, the possibility of environmental/food allergy takes on greater significance, and the approach is to manage clinical signs during the first month of the elimination diet. During the second month, discontinue the medication to verify the efficacy of the diet.

If the diet keeps the patient free of episodes, challenge the patient after the second month as previously explained.

If the animal relapses in the second month despite the diet, assume that this is an atopic-like dermatitis or an environmental allergy, for which there are two options: one is testing for specific IgE antibodies to provide immunotherapy; the other option is to use lifelong medication to control the signs. This will depend on the intensity and frequency of episodes. A range of drugs may be used, from occasional corticosteroids to long-term cyclosporine.

CLINICAL COURSE

The patient was stabilised by fogging the environment to eliminate juvenile fleas. Flea treatment was also strictly administered to control adult forms on the cat.

Treatment with dexamethasone 0.25 mg/cat/day was given for 5 days and then on alternating days for another 10 days. A strict elimination diet was also instituted.

Because the diet was ineffective, short-term treatment was recommenced with corticosteroids and cyclosporine 7 mg/kg/day (Fig. 3).

The future goal is to space out doses of cyclosporine until the minimum effective dose without corticosteroids is attained; corticosteroids should be reserved only for relapses.

Logically, other options exist depending on several factors, such as the use of antihistamines, palmitoylethanolamide, and other corticosteroids.

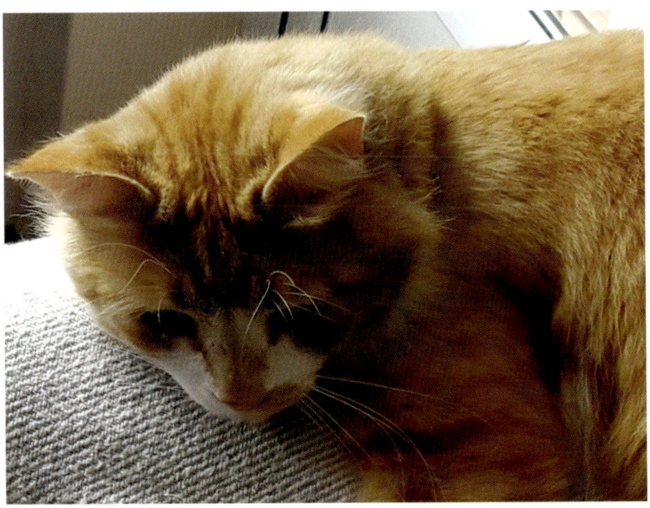

Figure 3. Condition of the patient 2 months after being stabilised.

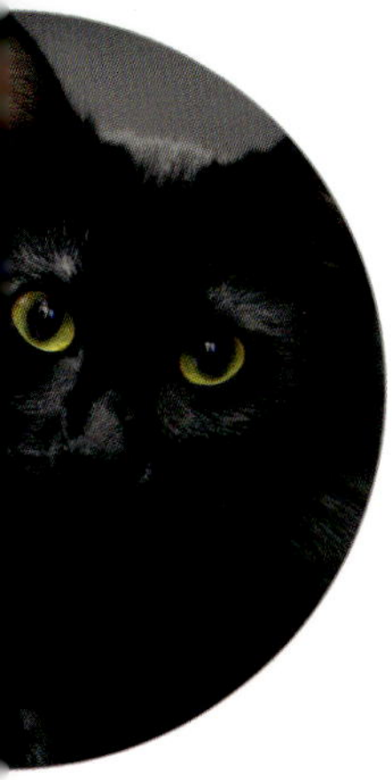

CHRONIC CASES

REFRACTORY ATOPY

This section shares observations from case studies of severely atopic dogs that have structural skin lesions because of their chronic signs and a lengthy history of complications; the disease may almost be thought of as autoimmune. In these cases, our experience and knowledge must come to the fore to make use of all treatment options in a fully individualised way (i.e. combinations and doses).

Drugs are designed for a majority of the population, which usually includes approximately 80 % of individuals. Nonetheless, there are always individual cases above or below the average that require different management, such as a higher or lower dose than that provided in a drug insert.

Recall that these chronic canine patients with refractory forms of the disease are generally suffering from severe xerosis, abnormal microbiota, and a high degree of pruritus that feed back into their clinical signs.

For this reason, we must find specific medications to control the signs and restore normal skin structure as much as possible. In short, we have to break the feedback loop of inflammation–pruritus–infection.

These patients generally have already undergone several treatments and diagnostic methods, and regardless of whether these were performed properly, in many cases the patient and owner have landed in a desperate situation.

The owners of these patients are understandably tired and discouraged by the disease; in this situation, veterinary surgeons must recover their trust by directly resolving signs and turning the situation around without worrying about diagnosing the exact primary disease.

The figures show canine patients with a pruritus score above 8, whose owners are often already familiar with all available drug treatments (Figs. 1–4).

To tackle these situations, it is important to consider the following very important points.

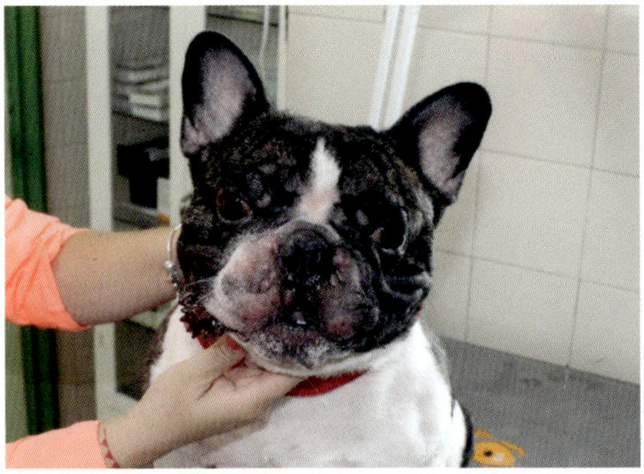

Figure 1. Severe facial inflammation in an atopic dog not responding to conventional treatments.

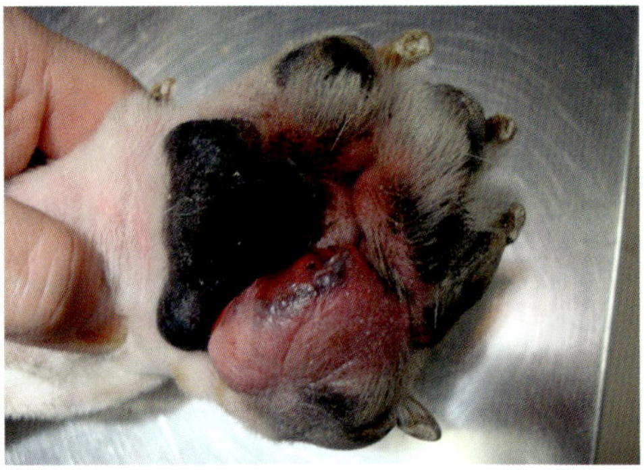

Figure 2. Interdigital inflammation due to compulsive licking.

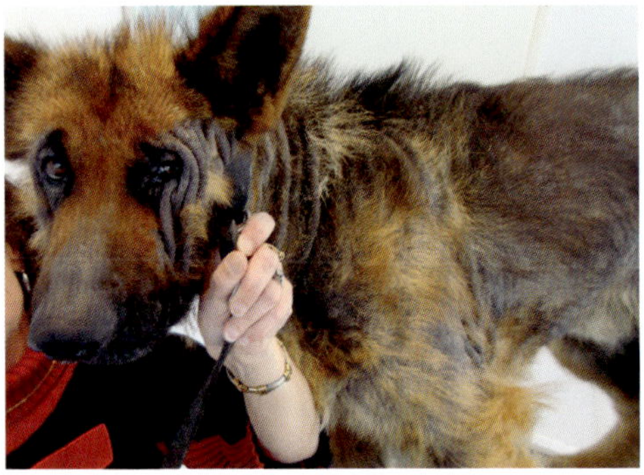

Figure 3. Patient with chronic microbial overgrowth and severe pruritus.

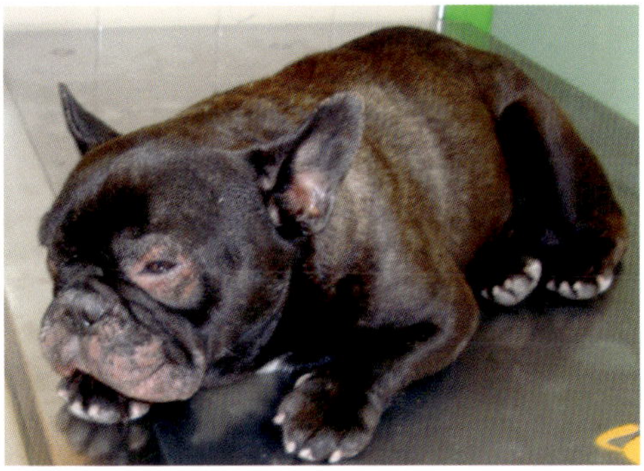

Figure 4. Patient with severe infected lesions due to uncontrolled pruritus.

INFORMATION FROM THE HISTORY

First of all, we must know all the medications used, how long each was administered for, and the doses. This is important because it will highlight the causes of resistance to treatment. This information will determine whether the problem is caused by insufficient treatment duration or by insufficient dosing. Failures can often arise from poorly compliant owners. However, recall that pharmacogenetics can mean that some individuals respond in a different way to treatment.

We must also know the details of the animal's environment and lifestyle. For example, if the animal's life is fully urban or if it is punctuated by intervals of rural life, etc.

THOROUGH EXAMINATION

In general, be very thorough to rule out underlying diseases that may predispose to treatment failure. For example, hypothyroid dogs, immunodeficient dogs with chronic pyoderma inherent to the breed (German Shepherd, Bull Terrier, etc.).

During the dermatological examination, it is very important to observe areas where microbial overgrowth would be most apparent, such as the interdigital spaces, ears, and the perianal and perioral areas (Fig. 5).

Special attention must also be paid to the distribution of body lesions in general and to strategically performing the most useful diagnostic tests for this patient. Adhesive tape and brushing are the initial tests to look for parasites and microbial overgrowth. Antibiotic sensitivity tests are also useful for patients who have already received many antibiotics.

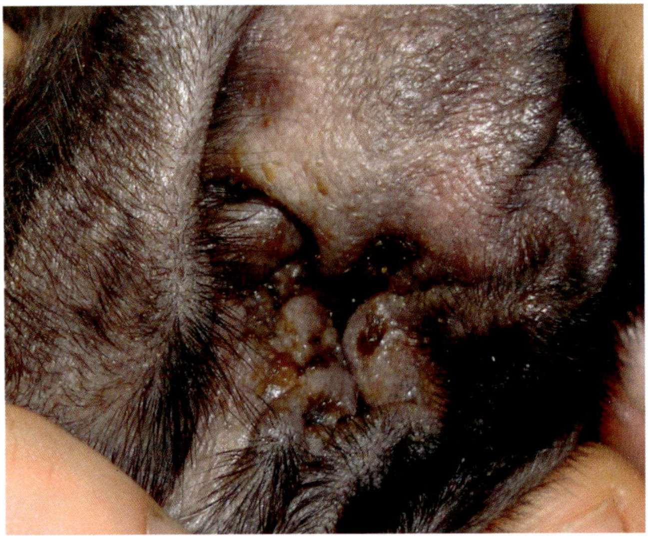

Figure 5. Ear with hyperplasia and excess wax.

If the test results, combined with the information obtained from the history, confirm that this is an uncontrolled atopic animal, we should develop the best treatment strategy specifically adapted to the animal and owner.

> **The aim is to develop a maintenance treatment to restore the skin structure and decrease the pruritus score below 5.**

We may have to combine several systemic and topical medications. This treatment must be adapted to the owner's financial capacity, compliance, and ability to handle the patient. For example, it is not easy for an owner to strictly comply with bathing a 90 kg Saint Bernard every two days. This animal must be very carefully dried and brushed to avoid mats that may trigger a new cycle of inflammation and pruritus; this recommendation is very difficult for the owner to fulfil.

If the history suggests that all the previous medication has been properly administered, the ideal step is referral of the case to a specialist. In general, a specialist has various resources to stabilise the animal and subsequently refer the case back to the patient's usual veterinary surgeon for monitoring and maintenance.

The treatment measures used in these cases might be labelled "last resort" and may include:

- Administering at or above the maximum the dose of medication under our care and supervision. Some individuals only respond to permanent high doses of a drug, and in these cases, we can combine with other drugs to enable lowering these doses. In all cases requiring prolonged high doses, we must follow patients closely with frequent rechecks. It is essential to follow the premise of "first do no harm", and veterinary surgeons should strive for a good quality of life for the patient and its owner, although this sometimes means deviating from the usual course (Fig. 6).
- Owners must always be notified of this exceptional management procedure.
- Antipruritogenic agents such as oclacitinib or cyclosporine may be combined with other drugs that boost their effects, such as corticosteroids.
- Lokivetmab may be a good baseline option that can be complemented with occasional administration of oclacitinib.
- The use of topical corticosteroids may enable the dose of certain systemic drugs to be reduced.

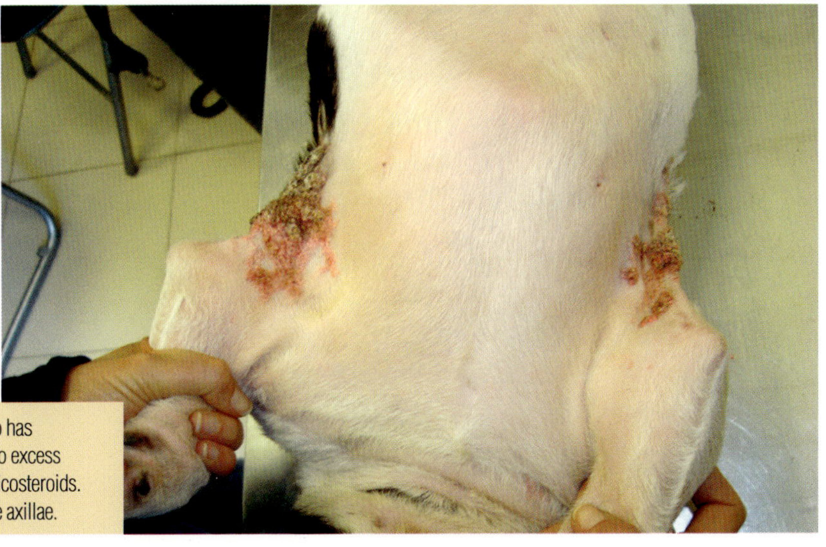

Figure 6. Dog who has decompensated due to excess administration of corticosteroids. Calcinosis cutis in the axillae.

- Nutraceuticals in high quality food products or long-term supplements, combined with frequent use of antiseptics and moisturisers in shampoos or sprays, usually help to improve the affected skin's condition.
- In uncontrolled animals positive for ectoparasites, consider a diet of wet food containing novel components or proteins for which the animal is negative on immunoglobulin serology.
- The patient's hair should be short to avoid accumulation of pollen or mites in the skin; wiping down the animal's haircoat with wet cloths will avoid the inflammation produced by harsh brushing with metal-bristled brushes.
- Do not dry with hot air after bathing so as not to dry out the skin.
- In severe cases, the use of immunosuppressant drugs can be considered, as long as the risk involved is understood.
- Control of microbiota by cleaning the interdigital spaces and mucocutaneous areas with antiseptic wipes may help to limit microbial overgrowth.
- Azole pulse therapy two days per week is commonly used to control *Malassezia*. Do not use antibiotics for pulse therapy.
- Overgrowth of bacteria and *Malassezia* in predisposed ears may be controlled with the periodic use of antiseptics or peptides.
- These patients must be followed carefully, perhaps quarterly. This monitoring consists of urine sediment and culture, abdominal ultrasound, and chest radiographs.

Finally, remember that in addition to the difficulty of finding the correct medication for the patient (which may require major effort by the owner), these situations are not usually static and we must be very attentive to correct doses or switch drugs if the situation so requires.

In these extremely severe cases, good communication between the dermatologist and regular vet is essential because the latter will bear the entire responsibility for the case under the advice and occasional follow-up by the specialist.

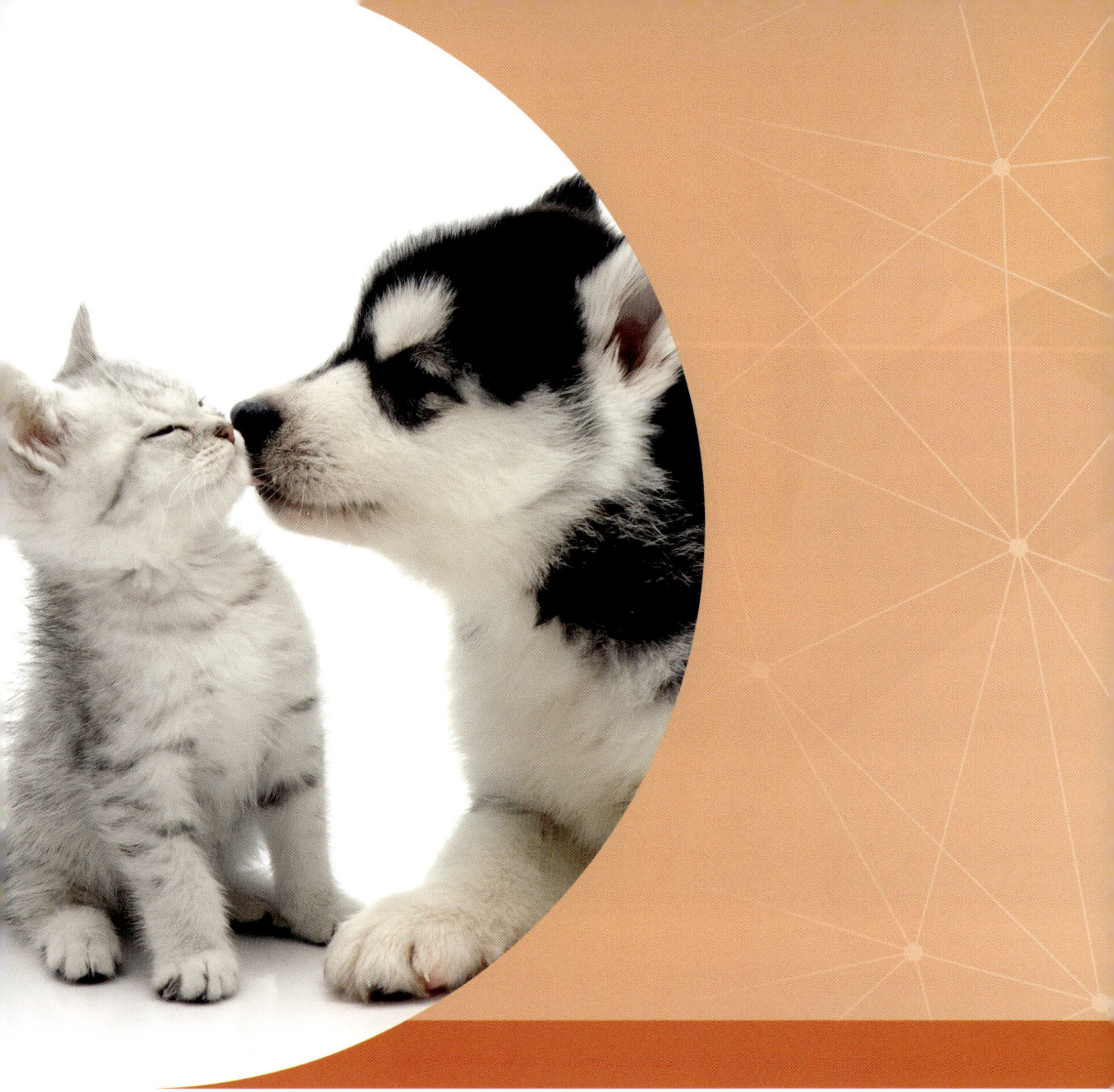

7

FURTHER INFORMATION

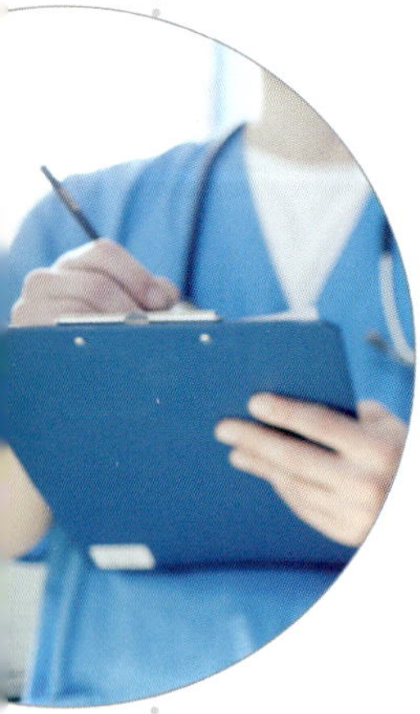

MOST COMMON COMPLICATIONS
IN DOGS WITH ALLERGY

This section will deal with the most common abnormalities in dogs with atopic dermatitis. Considering that these patients usually have deficiencies in skin structure, microbiota, and local defences, as well as excess production of pro-inflammatory interleukins and immunoglobulins that accompany hypersensitivity, complications are as follows:

CUTANEOUS
XEROSIS

Xerosis is dryness of the skin, mucosa, or conjunctiva. This characteristic of atopic skin is important in human medicine. In the last few years, based on prior studies in humans, canine dermatologists have confirmed that structural defects cause atopic canine skin to lose more water than normal because its abnormal structure impedes water retention. A deficiency in sphingosines and filaggrins causes water to evaporate more quickly and facilitates percutaneous ingress of allergens. Moreover, this structural defect goes hand-in-hand with abnormalities of the skin environment, with a consequent imbalance in the normal microbiota and substances that regulate it, such as certain fatty acids and peptides (Fig. 1).

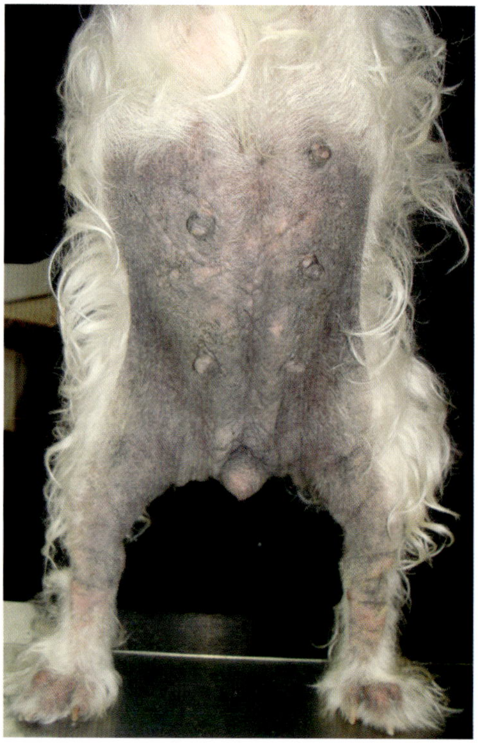

Figure 1. Significant xerosis in a dog with chronic atopic dermatitis.

All our knowledge to date supports the use of topical moisturising, hydrating and emollient treatments combined with microbiota-normalising agents such as antiseptics and microbiostatic substances. Treatment is also possible using proper nutrition together with dermoprotective components, which can be obtained through a high-end commercial diet or certain supplements.

Currently, a revolution in dermatological treatment and diagnosis means that new diagnostic possibilities and treatments for allergies are likely to arise in the near future. Monoclonal antibodies, antiparasitics, and antipruritogenic agents have evolved and significantly enhanced treatment possibilities. Thus, we must be diligent about diagnosis and avoid merely treating signs.

MOST COMMON TYPES OF ALLERGIC PYODERMA

BACTERIAL OVERGROWTH

Returning to the prior description of multifactorial skin deficiencies in the allergic dog, these patients usually have an imbalance in their skin's bacterial microbiota (Fig. 2). This usually has only a superficial impact, although the imbalance can reach the follicle or sebaceous gland and produce seborrhoea and rash, which later evolve into alopecia, lichenification, hyperpigmentation, and a characteristic musty smell. Sometimes the clinical signs are characterised by a greasy skin rather than by desquamation. The areas most commonly affected are usually the ventral neck, thorax, axillae, and groin. In severe cases, the abnormality may extend to the rest of the body, including interdigital spaces and the pinnae. The face may also be affected, inducing periocular and perioral signs.

This clinical picture is seen mainly in uncontrolled dogs with chronic disease whose owners have not yet dedicated sufficient attention or in cases where the veterinary clinician has not managed to get the situation under control.

Shampoo therapy and nutrition are essential to manage these patients who, depending on the severity of the case, may require varied supportive therapies ranging from oral or topical administration of essential fatty acids to topical application of antiseptics or antipruritogenic/anti-inflammatory agents such as oclacitinib or cyclosporine.

The use of spa therapy has only been investigated in terms of application of thermal clays to areas of pruritus or microbial overgrowth. This may permit reducing the dose of other medications.

> Corticosteroids may play an important role in severe cases requiring a more drastic reduction in inflammation.

Lokivetmab can also be used as a maintenance drug in controlled patients with a chronic predisposition to atopic allergic pruritus.

As outlined throughout this guide, the choice of treatment logically depends on the severity of the case, type of patient, and characteristics of the owner.

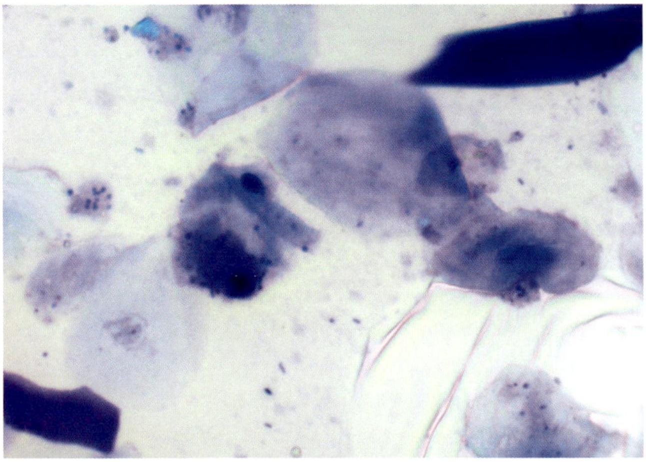

Figure 2. Cytology of bacterial overgrowth performed with adhesive tape.

PYOTRAUMATIC DERMATITIS

This is another kind of superficial pyoderma that, although generally benign, may be recurrent and extend deeper into the skin and become very painful. Certain breeds such as the Labrador and Saint Bernard are more predisposed to this condition, although no breed is immune (Fig. 3).

Its aetiopathogenesis is related to hyperacute onset of discomfort in a specific area of the body, usually the hind end or cheeks; despite often being related to the presence of fleas, its sudden onset may also be due to joint or rectal pain, otitis, or any other ear discomfort.

However, the veterinary surgeon is often unable to determine the exact cause of the problem and may find it simply consistent with an allergy.

Several treatments are available to prevent recurrence: use good ectoparasite prevention, dry the patient well after bathing, and keep the coat and skin clean and free of damage and parasites. Keep the hair as short as possible, brush gently, and avoid any kind of insect bite.

In animals with recurring pyotraumatic dermatitis of the hind end, consider that the hip joint may require NSAIDs.

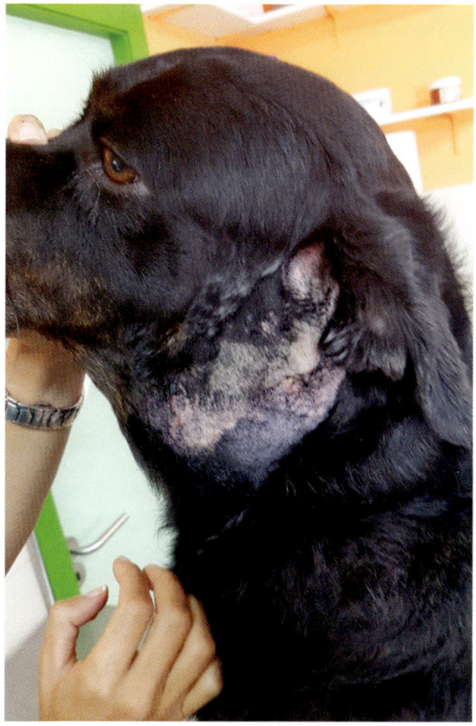

Figure 3. Classic subauricular pyotraumatic dermatitis resulting from ear pruritus.

In general, these cases require careful wound care, topical antiseptics, and, in some cases, corticosteroids or oclacitinib.

These conditions may worsen until furunculosis occurs. In these cases, systemic antibiotics must be used and corticosteroids must be avoided. Oclacitinib is a very good drug to prevent scratching of the affected area, regardless of how deep the condition is.

MUCOCUTANEOUS PYODERMA

Food allergens may play a significant role in allergic diseases such as canine atopic dermatitis; these are not food allergies per se but rather a combination of environmental and food allergies.

Many patients develop pruritus in areas of the gastrointestinal system such as the mouth and perianal area. This pruritus may lead to superficial infections, which in some cases may also extend to the edges of the nostrils and genital areas.

This type of pyoderma may also be associated with ocular dryness and lack of moisture of the nose and, in some cases, perioral contact dermatitis (Fig. 4).

Treatment depends on the severity, and although proper cleaning and application of antiseptics is often sufficient, systemic antibiotics may be necessary.

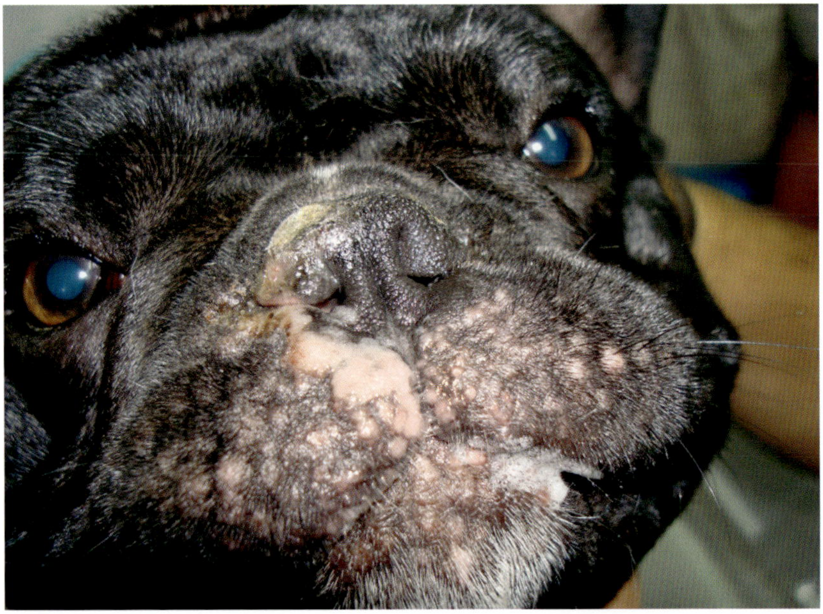

Figure 4. Mucocutaneous pyoderma. Note the cheilitis and infection in the perinasal area.

BACTERIAL FOLLICULITIS

In addition to conventional cases with lichenification, alopecia, and hyperpigmentation due to chronic microbial overgrowth, the most common pattern observed in atopic dogs is moth-eaten alopecia (Fig. 5).

This condition is more common in short-haired dogs, whose coat accentuates it. Bulldogs, Shar Peis, and Dalmatians are three of the most affected breeds.

> Bacterial folliculitis is very common and problematic in veterinary practice.

The initial differential diagnosis of bacterial folliculitis involves checking for *Demodex* and dermatophytes. These signs usually have a bacterial cause, and their response to antibiotics will confirm this.

The paradox is that most dogs with these signs are atopic. However, few of these patients have significant pruritus, and in some cases owners do not even consider pruritus a problem at all.

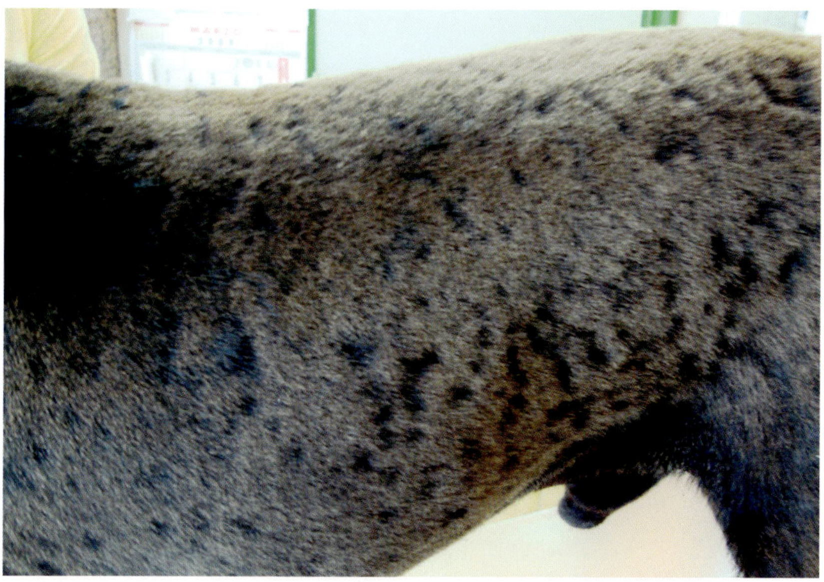

Figure 5. Classic moth-eaten appearance of bacterial folliculitis in the atopic dog.

Nonetheless, an in-depth investigation will verify that these patients respond to topical antiseptics and often oral antibiotics, but they also usually improve or go into remission when they are maintained on antipruritogenic agents. In these cases, the history can reveal certain behaviours related to pruritus (licking paws, rubbing themselves on surfaces for relief, etc).

Note that for a long time these alopecia-inducing signs were confused with dermatophytosis based on the incorrect conclusion that they improved when oral azoles were administered. This improvement could actually be accounted for by the anti-inflammatory action of these drugs.

DEEP PYODERMA

Individuals of certain breeds may be predisposed to deep pyoderma: German Shepherds, Bull Terriers and Staffordshire Terriers. This is because these breeds tend to develop furunculosis and cellulitis (for example, the German Shepherd is predisposed to immunodeficiency).

These may be a challenge for the veterinary clinician, who must not only control the acute disease but also provide management recommendations to the owner to avoid relapses (Fig. 6).

In the case of the German Shepherd, the frequent use of antiseptics, keeping the hair short, avoiding flies, offering a high quality diet, and administering immunomodulators may be very important. Many of these patients improve on cyclosporine because of its immunomodulatory effect that helps atopic dogs. A similar phenomenon occurs in the other short-haired breeds mentioned.

It is important to avoid traumas that trigger small injuries: avoid rugged terrain, hard floors, insects, and aggressive brushing.

In recurrent cases, culture and antibiotic sensitivity tests of affected dermis and hypodermis samples may be the best way to identify successful treatment. These samples may be derived from a biopsy placed in saline solution.

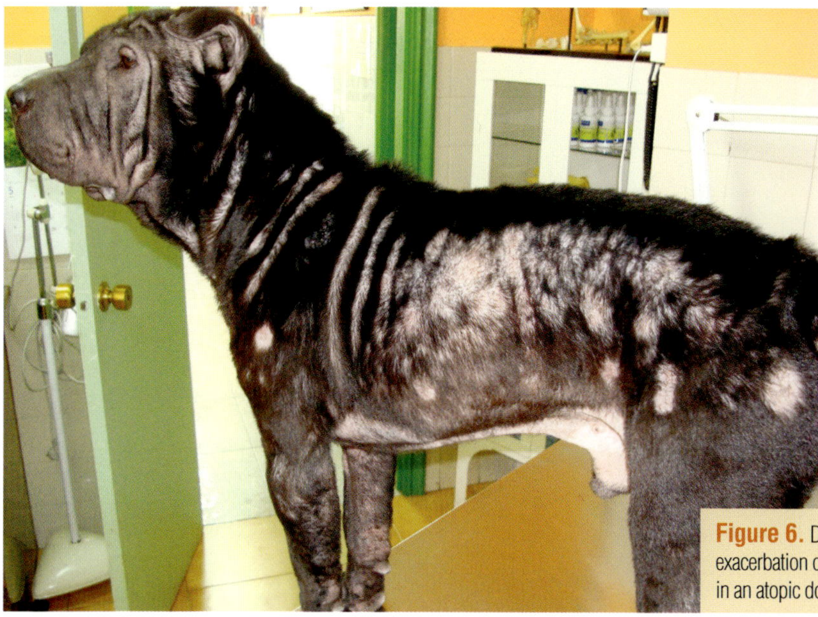

Figure 6. Deep pyoderma from exacerbation of bacterial folliculitis in an atopic dog.

OTITIS

Inflammation of the skin of the ear canal and its adnexa, which occurs in some allergic dogs, is the primary inciting factor for secondary bacterial agents and yeast to produce a complicated otitis.

Patients affected by this disease are generally predisposed to it, but various circumstances must coincide for it to develop. Some dogs suffer only from uncomplicated ear pruritus and erythema. However, some factors may favour ear infection: wet ears, stenosis of the canal, wax hypersecretion, or poor grooming practices such as plucking hairs. If the veterinary surgeon does not intervene properly in these cases or if otitis recurs frequently, certain characteristics of the ear canal environment may change, altering epithelial migration of the canal and making infections more difficult to cure (Fig. 7).

It is very important for owners of allergic patients to keep the ear canals clean and clear to avoid any interruption of progressive epithelial cell migration from inside to outside the ear.

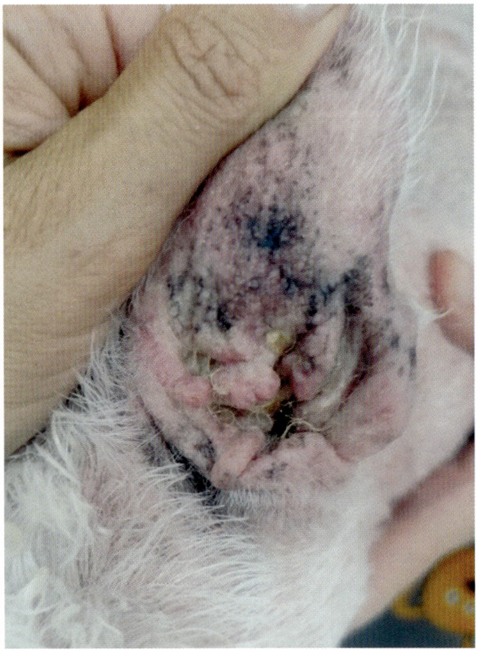

Figure 7. Severe abnormalities of the pinna in an atopic dog with recurrent otitis.

IMPORTANT POINTS ON OTITIS

1. Cleaning prior to treatment is essential.
2. Antibiotic sensitivity tests are required for cases of otitis involving bacilli or recurrent infections.
3. Treatment should be topical and applied in measured volumes, not numbers of drops.
4. Cytology will determine the onset and end of treatment.

MALASSEZIA OVERGROWTH

Much of the "Bacterial overgrowth" section applies to this point. Consider that overgrowth can be mixed, consisting of bacteria and *Malassezia* (Fig. 8).

We have to remember that this yeast is part of the normal microbiota of dog skin, but the abnormal skin environment in allergic animals can cause overgrowth or enzyme-induced hypersensitivity reactions.

Topical antiseptic treatments are essential (they are usually anti-yeast and antibacterial). They should be applied as frequently as needed. In some cases, the use of oral azoles or terbinafine may help to resolve signs more quickly. Certain very highly predisposed individuals will manage well with these systemic medications as pulse therapy, administered at weekends for example.

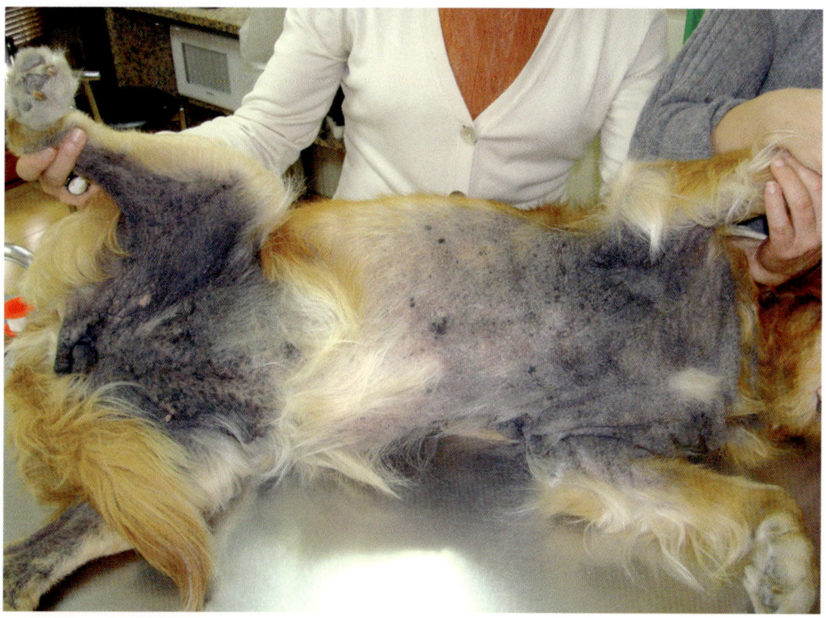

Figure 8. *Malassezia* overgrowth with hyperpigmentation and lichenification in an atopic dog.

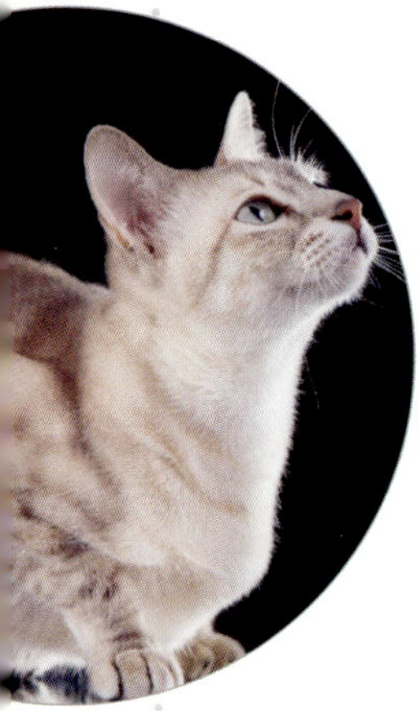

MOST COMMON
COMPLICATIONS
IN ALLERGIC CATS

The clinician's concern is completely different with cats than with dogs. Due to the specific characteristics of cat skin, pyoderma and *Malassezia* overgrowth are uncommon. These conditions occur, but much less often than in dogs and usually more as complications of the typical manifestations of allergy.

Remember the reaction patterns of allergic cats:

- Self-induced alopecia.
- Eosinophilic complex (granuloma, indolent plaque and ulcer).
- Head and neck dermatitis.
- Miliary dermatitis.

In cats, complications generally involve recurrences of these reactive processes or poor response to treatments.

> Pyoderma is usually less common than in dogs but is often a complication of allergic disease.

In cats, frequent licking caused by eosinophilic lesions or military dermatitis can lead to infections in plaque form. Indolent ulcer, generally found on the upper lip, usually contains superficial bacteria (Fig. 9).

Veterinary surgeons are familiar with frustrating facial clinical signs in cats and treatment-refractory self-induced alopecia.

In the case of eosinophilic plaques or granulomas, antibiotics may be necessary to treat bacterial complications (Fig. 10). In some cases the corticosteroid must be switched because of poor response to one drug. Many cats respond better to cyclosporine treatment.

TIP

It is essential to use flea preventive medication correctly. Moreover, rule out food allergies with diets (which may not always be palatable to the patient) and underscore the importance of environmental enrichment and use of pheromones to effect a change in behaviour.

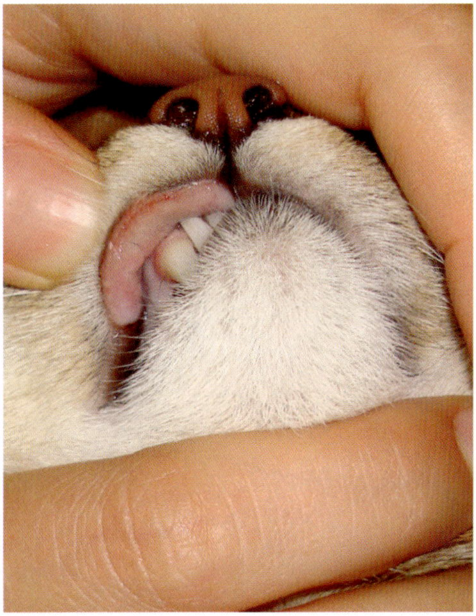

Figure 9. Indolent ulcer in an allergic cat.

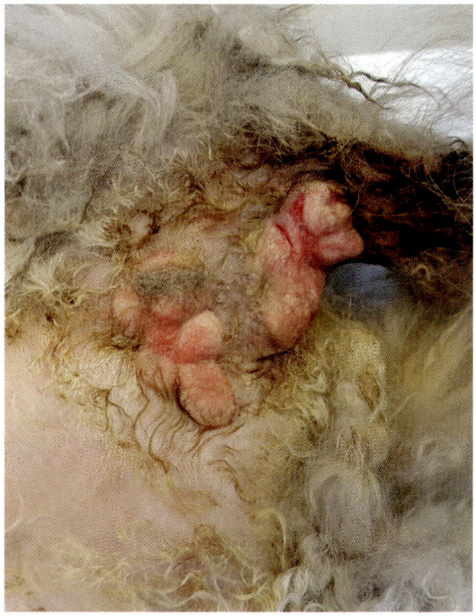

Figure 10. Severe eosinophilic granuloma in a Persian cat.

Cats are not as likely as dogs to develop iatrogenic Cushing's disease from corticosteroids. Nonetheless, we must use them with restraint. Other treatments that may help to control signs:

- Antihistamines.
- Palmitoylethanolamide.
- Topical corticosteroids.
- Cyclosporine.
- In some cases oclacitinib (too few studies to date).

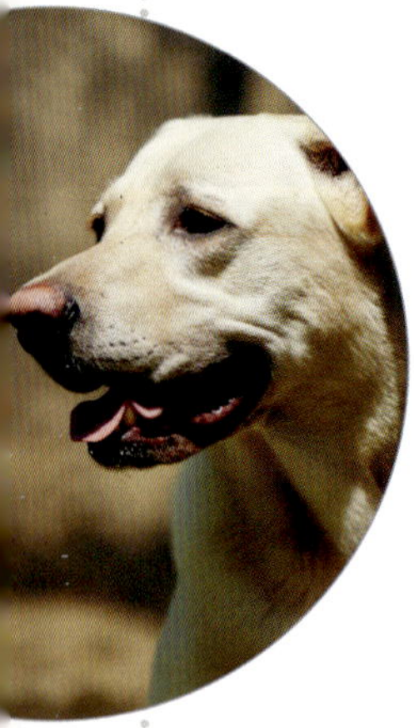

ENDOCRINE DISORDERS
AND ADVANCED AGE
AS AGGRAVATING FACTORS IN ALLERGIES

Some dogs have a mild allergic profile that enables them to lead a virtually normal life with almost total disease control, except for very sporadic skin episodes or otitis; however, they undergo typical changes with age that can disturb previously controlled clinical signs and lead to unprecedented episodes of allergy, otitis and pruritus.

These cases are often interpreted as dogs with late-onset allergy, but in reality they already had a mild disease that was aggravated by new factors.

Dogs become more likely to develop endocrine disorders such as hypothyroidism and Cushing's disease at 5 or 6 years old.

The allergic patient's predisposition to abnormalities of the microbiota, together with the skin manifestations of endocrine disorders such as xerosis, hyperpigmentation, diffuse alopecia, and metabolic abnormalities, mean that pyoderma is quite common.

Treatment of these imbalances allows the allergic patient to return to its previous state.

In senior patients, the skin's recovery capacity declines, along with changes in keratinocyte turnover and a decrease in immune function (Fig.11). As a consequence, allergies may be expressed much more intensely.

This condition can also occur in cats, mainly senior patients and those with hyperthyroidism. It is not uncommon to see senior cats with an eosinophilic reaction, mainly granuloma, that is much more refractory to treatment.

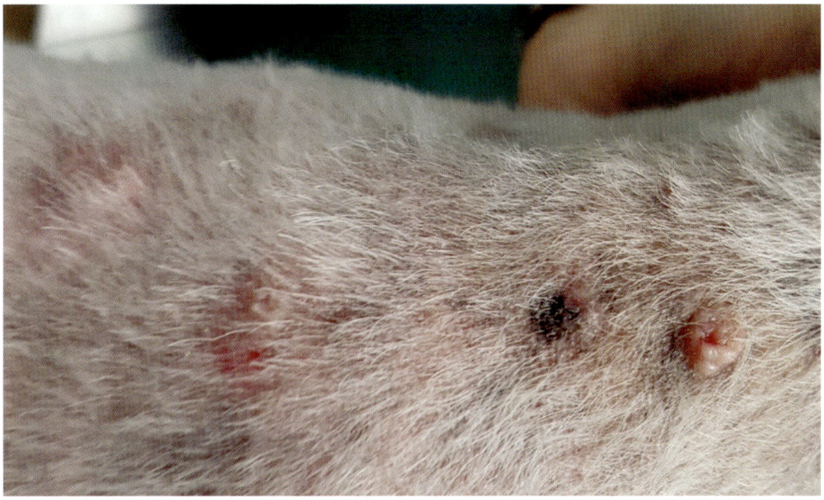

Figure 11. Appearance of skin outgrowths due to decreased turnover in an older dog.

ALPHABETICAL INDEX

M

O

P

S

T

BIBLIOGRAPHY

DAY, M.J. *Clinical Immunology of the Dog and Cat.* 2nd Edition. Manson 2012.

GONZÁLEZ, J., ORDEIX, L., MACHICOTE, G., YOTTI, C. *Formación Continuada Dermatología 2017.* AVEPA.

MACHICOTE, G. *Dermatología canina y felina. Manuales clínicos por especialidades.* Servet 2011.

MILLER, W., GRIFFIN, C.AND CAMPBELL, K. *Small Animal Dermatology.* 7th edition. Elsevier 2013.

OLIVRY, T., DEBOER, D.J., GRIFFIN, C.E., HALLIWELL, R.E., HILL, P.B., HILLIER, A., MARSELLA, R., SOUSA, C.A. The ACVD task force on canine atopic dermatitis: forewords and lexicon. *Vet Immunol Immunopathol,* 2001; 81(3–4):143–146.

OLIVRY, T., DEBOER, D.J., FAVROT, C., JACKSON, H.A., MUELLER, R.S., NUTTALL, T., PRÉLAUD; INTERNATIONAL TASK FORCE ON CANINE ATOPIC DERMATITIS. Treatment of canine atopic dermatitis: 2010 clinical practice guidelines from the International Task Force on Canine Atopic Dermatitis. *Vet Dermatol,* 2010; 21(3):233–248.

SANTORO, D., MARSELLA, R., PUCHEU-HASTON, C.M., EISENSCHENK, M.N., NUTTALL, T., BIZIKOVA, P. Review: Pathogenesis of canine atopic dermatitis: skin barrier and host-micro-organism interaction. *Vet Dermatol,* 2015; 26(2):84–e25.

RODRÍGUEZ, L., MANZUC, P. *Prurito canino: diagnóstico y tratamiento.* Intermédica 2014.

PHOTOGRAPHY
CREDITS

SHUTERSTOCK.COM
WilleeCole Photography: p. 13
VP Photo Studio: pp. 18, 23
michaeljung: pp. 20, 34
Eric Isselee: pp. 25, 26, 85
Ermolaev Alexander: pp. 27, 53
Ivonne Wierink: p. 30
Syda Productions: pp. 38, 40
Romaset: p. 44
Erik Lam: p. 53
Hadou: p. 54
Pressmaster: pp. 56, 58, 60, 110
Burdun Iliya: p. 64
Phensri Ngamsommitr: p. 68
Impact Photography: p. 73
Robert Neumann. p. 74
Budimir Jevtic: p. 78
nd3000: p. 80
Sebastian Kaulitzki: p. 82
135pixels: p. 83
didesign021: p. 90
Cosmin Manci: p. 94
Nikolai Tsvetkov: p. 98
Suzi Nelson: p. 101
ANURAK PONGPATIMET: p. 108
Anna Averianova: p. 120
Jaromir Chalabala: p. 122